SEXUALLY TRANSMITTED DISEASES

A Practical Guide

Symptoms, Diagnosis, Treatment, Prevention

Assembled and Edited

by

Robert J. Banis, Ph.D.

Science & Humanities Press

PO Box 7151

Chesterfield, MO 63006-7151

Publication Date, February, 2006
ISBN 1-888725-58-3

Library of Congress Cataloging-in-Publication Data
Banis, Robert J.
 Sexually transmitted diseases : a practical guide : symptoms, diagnosis, treatment, prevention / assembled and edited by Robert J. Banis.-- 2nd ed.
  p. cm.
 Includes bibliographical references.
 ISBN 1-888725-58-3 (alk. paper)
 1. Sexually transmitted diseases--Popular works. I. Title.
RC200.2.B36 2006
616.95'1--dc22   2006006062

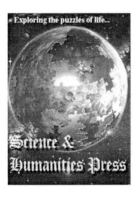

Science & Humanities Press
PO Box 7151
Chesterfield, MO 63006-7151
sciencehumanitiespress.com

Foreword

This book is a compendium of information from several sources, primarily derived from official documents of the United States National Institute of Arthritis and Infectious Diseases (NIAID). References to NIAID work and additional resources were left intact to facilitate further study.

The text was edited to combine documents and reduce overlap and repetition.

This book is part of a continuing effort to increase accessibility of information which is in the public domain and so permission is granted to copy it for nonprofit educational use. Copyright does not apply to US Government-derived parts. There is a quantity discount schedule for educational and healthcare professionals.

Although derived from official and expert sources, it should not be construed as definitive medical advice. The purpose is to raise awareness so that you will know where to go for help.

Please consult with public health facilities and your own private physician about personal health issues.

Robert J. Banis, Ph.D.

St. Louis, Missouri ~ January, 2006

Table of Contents

Sexually Transmitted Diseases

A Practical Guide

Sexually Transmitted Diseases—
Five Key Points:

Sexually transmitted diseases (STDs), once called venereal diseases, are among the most common infectious diseases in the United States today. More than 20 STDs have now been identified, and they affect up to 19 million men and women in this country each year. The annual comprehensive cost of STDs in the United States is estimated to be well in excess of $13 billion.

Understanding the basic facts about STDs--the ways in which they are spread, their common symptoms, and how they can be treated--is the first step toward prevention.

What are some of these basic facts?

It is important to understand at least five key points about all STDs in this country today:

STDs affect men and women of all backgrounds and economic levels. They are most prevalent among teenagers and young adults. Nearly two thirds of all STDs occur in people younger than 25 years of age.

The incidence of STDs is rising, in part because in the last few decades, young people have become sexually active earlier yet are marrying later. In addition, divorce is more common. The net result is that sexually active people today are more likely to have multiple sex partners during their lives and are potentially at risk for developing STDs.

Many STDs initially cause no symptoms, particularly in women. When symptoms develop, they may be confused with those of other diseases not transmitted through sexual contact. However, even when an STD causes no symptoms, a person who is infected may be able to pass the disease on to a sex partner. That is why many doctors recommend periodic testing for people who have more than one sex partner.

Health problems caused by STDs tend to be more severe and more frequent for women than for men, in part because the frequency of asymptomatic infection means that many women do not seek care until serious problems have developed. Some STDs can spread into the uterus (womb) and fallopian tubes to cause pelvic inflammatory disease (PID), which in turn is a major cause of both infertility and ectopic (tubal) pregnancy. The latter can be fatal. STDs in women may also be associated with cervical cancer. One STD, human papillomavirus infection (HPV), can result in genital warts, but can also lead to cervical and other genital cancers; the relationship between other STDs and cervical cancer is not yet clear. STDs can be passed from a mother to her baby before or during birth; some of these infections of the newborn can be cured easily, but others may cause a baby to be permanently disabled or even die.

When diagnosed and treated early, almost all STDs can be treated effectively. Some organisms, such as certain forms of gonococci, have become resistant to the drugs used to treat them and now require newer types of antibiotics. The most serious STD for which no cure now exists is acquired immunodeficiency syndrome (AIDS), a fatal viral infection of the immune system. Experts believe that having STDs other than AIDS increases one's risk for becoming infected with the AIDS virus.

There are very active research programs focused on finding better methods of diagnosis and more effective treatments, as well as producing vaccines that could one day ensure that STDs, like many other infectious diseases, no longer pose serious threats to health.

What Can You Do to Prevent STDs?

The best way to prevent STDs is to not have sexual intercourse. If you decide to be sexually active, there are things that you can do to reduce your risk of developing an STD.

- Be direct and frank about asking a new sex partner whether he or she has an STD, has been exposed to one, or has any unexplained physical symptoms.

- Learn to recognize the physical signs of STDs and inspect a sex partner's body, especially the genital area, for sores, rashes, or discharges.

- Don't have sex if your partner has signs or symptoms of STDs. Urge him/her to get medical attention as soon as possible.

Use a condom (rubber) during sexual intercourse and learn to use it correctly. Diaphragms may also reduce the risk of transmission of some STDs. Although there is some laboratory evidence that spermicides can kill STD organisms, scientists are still evaluating the usefulness of spermicides in preventing STDs. Some studies have found that frequent use of spermicides (more than three times a week) may cause vaginal inflammation.

Anyone who is sexually active with someone other than a long-term monogamous partner should:

- Have regular checkups for STDs even in the absence of symptoms. These tests can be done during a routine visit to the doctor's office.

- Learn the common symptoms of STDs. Seek medical help immediately if any suspicious symptoms develop, even if they are mild.

Anyone diagnosed as having an STD should:

- Notify all recent sex partners and urge them to get a checkup.

- Follow the doctor's orders and complete the full course of medication prescribed. A follow-up test to ensure that the infection has been cured is often an important final step in treatment.
- Avoid all sexual activity while being treated for an STD.

Sometimes people are too embarrassed or frightened to ask for help or information. Most STDs are readily treated, and the earlier a person seeks treatment and warns sex partners about the disease, the less likely that the disease will do irreparable physical damage, be spread to others or, in the case of a woman, be passed on to a newborn baby.

Private Doctors, local health departments, and STD and family planning clinics have information about STDs. In addition, the American Social Health Association (ASHA) provides free information and keeps lists of clinics and private doctors who provide treatment for people with STDs. ASHA has a website at http://www.ashastd.org/index.cfm.

Research may someday result in detection methods, medications and vaccines that could make STDs less of a health risk. Modern antibiotics have done much to improve treatment.

It is up to each individual to learn more about STDs and then make choices about how to minimize the risk of acquiring these diseases and spreading them to others. Knowledge of STDs, as well as honesty and openness with sex partners and with one's doctor, can be very important in reducing the incidence and complications of sexually transmitted diseases.

Diseases That May Be Transmitted Sexually and the Organisms Responsible

Disease	Organism(s)
Acquired Immunodeficiency Syndrome (AIDS)	Human immunodeficiency virus
Bacterial vaginosis	Bacteroides Gardnerella
vaginalis Mobiluncus spp.	Mycoplasma hominis Ureaplasma urealyticum
Chancroid	Haemophilus ducreyi
Chlamydial infections	Chlamydia trachomatis
Cytomegalovirus infections	Cytomegalovirus
Enteric infections	Hepatitis A Hepatitis A virus
Amebiasis	Entamoeba histolytica
(protozoan)	Giardia lamblia (protozoan)
Genital herpes	Herpes simplex virus
Genital (venereal) warts	Human papillomavirus
Gonorrhea	Neisseria gonorrhoeae
Granuloma inguinale (donovanosis)	Calymmatobacterium granulomatis
Group B streptococcal infections	Group B-hemolytic streptococcus
Leukemia/Lymphoma/ Myelopathy	HTLV-I and II
Lymphogranuloma Venereum	Chlamydia trachomatis
Molluscum contagiosum	Molluscum contagiosum virus
Pubic lice	Phthirus pubis
Scabies	Sarcoptes scabiei
Syphilis	Treponema pallidum
Trichomoniasis	Trichomonas vaginalis
Vaginal yeast infections	Candida albicans
Viral hepatitis	Hepatitis A, B, C, D viruses

Trends in Reportable Sexually Transmitted Diseases in the United States

National Surveillance Data for Chlamydia, Gonorrhea, and Syphilis

Sexually transmitted diseases (STDs) remain a major public health challenge in the United States. While substantial progress has been made in preventing, diagnosing, and treating certain STDs in recent years, CDC estimates that 19 million new infections occur each year, almost half of them among young people ages 15 to 24.[1] In addition to the physical and psychological consequences of STDs, these diseases also exact a tremendous economic toll. Direct medical costs associated with STDs in the United States are estimated at $13 billion annually.[2]

These data are presented in great detail in the CDC's report, **Sexually Transmitted Disease Surveillance 2004** (available at www.CDC.gov/STD/stats).

Although they are useful for examining overall trends and trends among populations at risk, they represent only a small proportion of the true national burden of STDs. Many cases of notifiable STDs go undiagnosed, and some highly prevalent viral infections, such as human papillomavirus and genital herpes, are not reported at all so we can only roughly estimate their prevalence.

Chlamydia: Expanded Screening Efforts Result in More Reported Cases, But Majority of Infections Remain Undiagnosed

Chlamydia remains the most commonly reported infectious disease in the United States. In 2004, 929,462 chlamydia diagnoses were reported, up from 877,478 in 2003. Even so, most chlamydia cases go undiagnosed. It is estimated that there are approximately 2.8 million new cases of chlamydia in the United States each year.[1]

The national rate of reported chlamydia in 2004 was 319.6 cases per 100,000 population, an increase of 5.9 percent from 2003 (301.7). The increases in reported cases and rates likely reflect the continued expansion of screening efforts and increased use of more sensitive diagnostic tests, rather than an actual increase in new infections.

Impact on Women

Women, especially young women, are hit hardest by chlamydia. Studies have found that chlamydia is more common among young women than young men, and the long-term consequences of untreated disease for women are much more severe. The chlamydia case rate for females in 2004 was 3.3 times higher than for males (485.0 vs. 147.1). However, much of this difference reflects the fact that women are far more likely to be screened than men. Females ages 15 to 19 had the highest chlamydia rate (2,761.5), followed by females ages 20 to 24 (2,630.7). African-American women are also disproportionately impacted by chlamydia. In 2004, the rate of reported chlamydia among black females (1,722.3) was more than 7.5 times that of white females (226.6). Because case reports do not provide a complete account of the burden of disease, researchers also evaluate chlamydia prevalence in subgroups of the population to better estimate the true extent of the disease. For example, data from chlamydia screening in family planning clinics across the United States indicates that roughly 6 percent of 15- to 24-year-old females in these settings are infected.

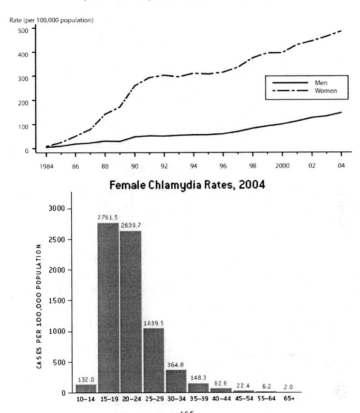

Chlamydia - Rates by sex: United States, 1984-2004

Rate (per 100,000 population)

Men
Women

Female Chlamydia Rates, 2004

Importance of Screening

Because chlamydia is most common among young women, CDC recommends annual chlamydia screening for sexually active women under age 26, as well as older women with risk factors such as new or multiple sex partners.5 Data from a study in a managed care setting suggest that chlamydia screening and treatment can reduce incidence of PID by over 50 percent.6 Unfortunately, many sexually active young women are not being tested for chlamydia, in part reflecting a lack of awareness among some providers and limited resources for screening.5, 7 recent research has shown that a simple change in clinical procedures — coupling chlamydia tests with routine Pap testing — can sharply increase the proportion of sexually active young women screened.8 Stepping up screening efforts is critical to preventing the serious health consequences of this infection, particularly infertility.

While screening is critical for sexually active young women, improved testing and treatment among men could help reduce transmission to women. The availability of urine tests for chlamydia may be contributing to increased detection of the disease in men, and consequently the rising rates of reported chlamydia in men in recent years (from 99.6 in 2000 to 147.1 in 2004).

Health Consequences of Chlamydia

Chlamydia is a bacterial infection that can easily be cured with antibiotics, but it is usually asymptomatic and often undiagnosed. Untreated, it can cause severe health consequences for women, including pelvic inflammatory disease (PID), ectopic pregnancy, and infertility. Up to 40 percent of females with untreated chlamydia infections develop PID, and 20 percent of those may become infertile.[3] In addition, women infected with chlamydia are up to five times more likely to become infected with HIV, if exposed.[4] Complications from chlamydia among men are relatively uncommon, but may include epididymitis and urethritis, which can cause pain, fever, and in rare cases, sterility.

Gonorrhea: Disease Rate Falls to Historic Low but Drug Resistance on the Rise

Gonorrhea is the second most commonly reported infectious disease in the United States, with 330,132 cases reported in 2004. From a high of 467.7 cases per 100,000 population reported in 1975, the U.S. gonorrhea rate fell to 113.5 in 2004 (a 76% decline) — the lowest recorded level since reporting began in 1941. More recently, from 2003 to 2004, the rate fell 1.5 percent (from 115.2 cases per 100,000 population to 113.5). Like chlamydia, however, gonorrhea is substantially under diagnosed and under reported, and approximately twice as many new infections are estimated to occur each year as are reported.[1]

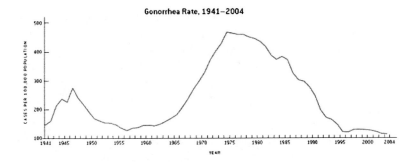

Gonorrhea Rate, 1941–2004

Racial Disparities Persist

African Americans remain the group most heavily affected by gonorrhea. While the rate of gonorrhea among blacks fell 3.0 percent from 2003 to 2004, the reported 2004 rate per 100,000 population for blacks (629.6) was 19 times greater than for whites (33.3). In 2003, the rate for blacks was 20 times higher than the rate for whites.

American Indians/Alaska Natives had the second-highest gonorrhea rate in 2004 (117.7, up 14.8% from 2003), followed by Hispanics (71.3, up 2.3% from 2003), whites (33.3, up 2.1% from 2003), and Asians/Pacific Islanders (21.4, down 3.2% from 2003).

Ethnic minorities in the United States have traditionally had higher rates of reported gonorrhea and other STDs, in part a reflection of limited access to quality health care, poverty, and higher background prevalence of disease in these populations.

Drug Resistance Increasing In Communities across the United States

Drug resistance is an increasingly important concern in the treatment and prevention of gonorrhea.10 CDC monitors trends in gonorrhea drug resistance through the Gonococcal Isolate Surveillance Project (GISP), which tests gonorrhea samples ("isolates") from the first 25 men with urethral gonorrhea attending STD clinics each month in sentinel clinics across the United States (28 cities in 2004).[11]

Overall, 6.8 percent of gonorrhea isolates tested through GISP in 2004 demonstrated resistance to fluoroquinolones, a leading class of antibiotics used to treat the disease, compared to 4.1 percent in 2003 and 2.2 percent in 2002. Resistance is especially worrisome among men who have sex with men (MSM), where resistance was eight times higher than among heterosexuals (23.8% vs. 2.9%).

In April 2004, CDC recommended that fluoroquinolones no longer be used as treatment for gonorrhea among MSM. Fluoroquinolones are also not recommended to treat gonorrhea in anyone in California and Hawaii, where fluoroquinolone-resistant cases have been widespread for several years. Outside of these states in 2004, 17.8 percent of gonorrhea isolates among MSM were resistant to fluoroquinolones, while resistance among heterosexuals remained low at 1.3 percent.

Health Consequences of Gonorrhea

While gonorrhea is easily cured, untreated cases can lead to serious health problems. Among women, gonorrhea is a major cause of PID, which can lead to chronic pelvic pain, ectopic pregnancy, and infertility. In men, untreated gonorrhea can cause epididymitis, a painful condition of the testicles that can result in infertility. In addition, studies suggest that presence of gonorrhea infection makes an individual three to five times more likely to acquire HIV, if exposed.[9]

Syphilis: Cases Increase for Fourth Consecutive Year

The rate of primary and secondary (P&S) syphilis — the most infectious stages of the disease — decreased throughout the 1990s, and in 2000 reached an all-time low. However, over the past four years the syphilis rate in the United States has been increasing. Between 2003 and 2004 alone, the national P&S syphilis rate increased 8 percent, from 2.5 to 2.7 cases per 100,000 population; during this time, reported P&S cases in the United States increased from 7,177 to 7,980.

Overall, increases in P&S syphilis rates between 2000 and 2004 were observed only among men. The rate of P&S syphilis among males rose 81 percent between 2000 and 2004 (from 2.6 to 4.7), and 11.9 percent between 2003 (4.2) and 2004. Notably, in 2004 — for the first time in over 10 years — the rate among females did not decrease, remaining at 0.8. Between 2003 and 2004, the rate of congenital syphilis (i.e., transmission from mother to child) decreased 17.8 percent (from 10.7 to 8.8 per 100,000 live births), likely reflecting the substantial reduction in syphilis among women that has occurred over the past decade.

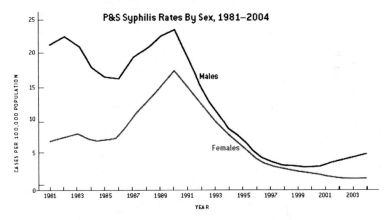

Rising Rate Driven By Cases among Men

Increasing cases of P&S syphilis among MSM are believed to be largely responsible for the overall increases in the national syphilis rate observed since 2000. Until very recently, CDC has not collected data by risk group. However, the male-to-female ratio for P&S syphilis has risen steadily between 2000 and 2004 (from 1.5 to 5.9), suggesting increased syphilis transmission among MSM. This increase occurred among all racial and ethnic groups. Additionally, CDC estimates that MSM comprised 64 percent of P&S syphilis cases in 2004, up from 5 percent in 1999.[12]

Recent Declines among African Americans Possibly Reversing

In 2004, the P&S syphilis rate among blacks increased for the first time in more than a decade — 16.9 percent from 2003 to 2004 (from 7.7 to 9.0), with the most significant increases among black men. Between 2003 and 2004, the syphilis rate among black males increased 22.6 percent (from 11.5 to 14.1), while the rate among black women rose 2.4 percent (from 4.2 to 4.3). In addition, the male-to-female ratio for blacks rose from 2.7 in 2003 to 3.3 in 2004, suggesting increases among black MSM.

Racial gaps in syphilis rates are narrowing, with rates in 2004 5.6 times higher among blacks than among whites, a substantially lower differential than in 2000, when the rate among blacks was 24 times greater than among whites. This narrowing reflects both declining disease rates among African Americans and the significant increases among white men in recent years. Continued progress in eliminating this disease will require an ongoing commitment to syphilis education, testing, and treatment in all populations affected.

Urban Areas Bear Greatest Syphilis Burden

Syphilis remains a public health problem in metropolitan areas with large populations of MSM. For the third consecutive year, San Francisco had the highest P&S rate of any U.S. city in 2004 (45.9). Other leading cities include Atlanta, Georgia (34.6); Baltimore, Maryland (33.2); New Orleans, Louisiana (16.4); St Louis, Missouri (14.1); Detroit, Michigan (13.5); Washington, D.C. (12.2); Dallas, Texas (11.6); Jersey City, New Jersey (10.8); and Chicago, Illinois (9.7).

Health Consequences of Syphilis

Syphilis, a genital ulcerative disease, is highly infectious, but easily curable in its early (primary and secondary) stages. If untreated, it can lead to serious long-term complications, including nerve, cardiovascular, and organ damage, and even death. Congenital syphilis can cause stillbirth, death soon after birth, and physical deformity and neurological complications in children who survive. Syphilis, like many other STDs, facilitates the spread of HIV, increasing transmission of the virus at least two- to five-fold.[13]

References

1 Weinstock H, Berman S, Cates W. Sexually transmitted diseases among American youth: incidence and prevalence estimates, 2000. Perspectives on Sexual and Reproductive Health 2004;36(1):6-10.

2 HW Chesson, JM Blandford, TL Gift, G Tao, KL Irwin. The estimated direct medical cost of STDs among American youth, 2000. Abstract P075. 2004 National STD Prevention Conference. Philadelphia, PA. March 8-11, 2004.

3 Hillis SD and Wasserheit JN. Screening for Chlamydia — A Key to the Prevention of Pelvic Inflammatory Disease. New England Journal of Medicine 1996;334(21):1399-1401.

4 CDC. Press Release: New CDC treatment guidelines critical to preventing consequences of sexually transmitted diseases. May 9, 2002.

5 CDC. Sexually Transmitted Disease Surveillance, 2004. Atlanta, GA: U.S. Department of Health and Human Services, September 2005.

6 Scholes D et al. Prevention of Pelvic Inflammatory Disease by Screening for Cervical Chlamydial Infection. New England Journal of Medicine 1996; 334(21):1362-1366.

7 CDC. Chlamydia screening among sexually active young female enrollees of health plans — United States, 1999 – 2001. Morbidity and Mortality Weekly Report 2004;53(42):983-985.

8 Burstein G et al. Chlamydia screening in a health plan before and after a national performance measure introduction. Obstetrics & Gynecology 2005;106(2):327-334.

9 Fleming DT and Wasserheit JN. From epidemiological synergy to public health policy and practice: the contribution of other sexually transmitted diseases to sexual transmission of HIV infection. Sexually Transmitted Infections 1999;75:3-17.

10 CDC. Increases in fluoroquinolone-resistant Neisseria gonorrhoeae among men who have sex with men — United States, 2003, and revised recommendations for gonorrhea treatment, 2004. Morbidity and Mortality Weekly Report 2004;53(16):335-338.

11 CDC. Gonococcal Isolate Surveillance Project. Available at: www.cdc.gov/std/gisp.

12 CDC. Unpublished data.

13 CDC. HIV Prevention Through Early Detection and Treatment of Other Sexually Transmitted Diseases — United States Recommendations of the Advisory Committee for HIV and STD Prevention. Morbidity and Mortality Weekly Report 1998; 47(RR-12):1-24.

Hepatitis

Hepatitis is an inflammation of the liver caused by certain viruses and other factors, such as alcohol abuse, some medications, and trauma. Its various forms affect millions of Americans. Although many cases of hepatitis are not a serious threat to health, the disease can become chronic (long-lasting) and can sometimes lead to liver failure and death.

Cause

There are four major types of viral hepatitis:

Hepatitis A, caused by infection with the hepatitis A virus, is usually a mild disease that does not become chronic. The virus is sometimes passed on through sexual practices involving oral-anal contact. It is most commonly spread by food and water contamination

Hepatitis B, caused by infection with the hepatitis B virus (HBV), may be mild or severe, acute or chronic. HBV is most commonly passed on to a sexual partner during intercourse, especially during anal sex. Because the disease is not easily spread, persons with HBV should not worry about spreading it through casual contact such as shaking hands or sharing a workspace or bathroom facility.

Each year, an estimated 300,000 persons in the United States become infected with HBV. Hepatitis B is most commonly transmitted by sharing drug needles, by engaging in high-risk sexual behavior, from a mother to her newborn, and in the health care setting.

Non-A, non-B hepatitis is primarily caused by the hepatitis C virus (HCV). Although generally a mild condition, it is much more likely than hepatitis B to lead to chronic liver disease. HCV appears to be spread through sexual contact as well as through sharing drug needles. Sexual spread, however, is inefficient and much less than that for HBV or the AIDS virus (HIV). With the advent of new tests to screen blood donors, a very small percentage of persons with HCV currently become infected through blood transfusions. The hepatitis E virus causes another type of non-A, non-B hepatitis. This virus is principally spread through contaminated water in areas with poor sanitation. This form of hepatitis does not occur in the U.S. and is not known to be passed on through sexual contact.

Delta hepatitis occurs only in people who already are infected with HBV. A potentially severe disease, it is caused by a virus (HDV) that can produce disease only when HBV is also present. Most cases occur among people who are frequently exposed to blood and blood products, such as people with hemophilia. Small-scale epidemics have occurred among injection drug users who share contaminated needles.

Experts believe that HDV may be sexually transmitted, but further research is needed to provide more specific evidence.

Transmission

HBV, HCV, and HDV can be spread in the following ways:

- Having sexual intercourse with an infected person without using a condom.
- Sharing drug needles among users of injected street drugs.
- Needle-stick accidents among health-care workers.
- Mother-to-child transmission of HBV during birth.

Transfusions. Until recently, blood transfusions were the most frequent cause of hepatitis C. Blood banks in the United States now screen donated blood for HBV and HCV and discard any blood that appears to be infected. Therefore, the risk of acquiring hepatitis from these viruses is very low in the U.S. and in other countries where blood is similarly tested. Tests to screen blood for HBV will also screen out HDV.

Personal contact with an infected person. HBV, HCV, and HDV sometimes spread when household members unknowingly come in contact with virus-infected blood or body fluids--most probably through cuts and scrapes or by sharing personal items such as razors and toothbrushes. While it is possible to become infected by contact with saliva, blood and semen remain the major sources of infection.

Symptoms

Many people infected with viral hepatitis have no symptoms. For example, about one-third of people infected with HBV have a completely "silent" disease. When symptoms are present, they may be mild or severe. The most common early symptoms are mild fever, headache, muscle aches, fatigue, loss of appetite, nausea, vomiting, or diarrhea. Later symptoms may include dark and foamy urine and pale feces; abdominal pain; and yellowing of the skin and whites of the eyes (jaundice).

About 15 to 20 percent of patients develop short-term arthritis-like problems as part of a more severe case of hepatitis B. Another one-third of those with hepatitis B develop only mild flu-like symptoms without jaundice. Very severe (fulminant) hepatitis B is rare, but life-threatening. Early signs of fulminant hepatitis, such as personality changes and agitated behavior, require immediate medical attention.

Some people infected with HBV or HCV become chronic carriers of the virus, although they may have no symptoms. There are an estimated 1.5 million HBV carriers in the U.S. and 300 million carriers worldwide. Children are at greatest risk. About 90 percent of babies who become infected at birth with HBV, and up to half of youngsters who are infected before age 5, become chronic carriers. It is estimated that there are between 2 and 5 million HCV chronic carriers. At least half of all HCV carriers will develop chronic liver disease, regardless of whether or not they have symptoms.

Diagnosis

Hepatitis B. Several types of blood tests can detect signs of HBV even before symptoms develop. These tests measure liver function and identify HBV antigens (proteins of the virus) or antibodies (proteins produced by the body in response to the virus) in the blood.

18

Tests for hepatitis B include:

Hepatitis B Surface Antigen (HBsAg). Most people with acute hepatitis B have HBsAg in their blood before symptoms develop. As a person recovers from the illness, HBsAg disappears. If it is still present 6 months after infection, it may indicate that a person has developed chronic hepatitis or may be a symptomless carrier of the virus. HBsAg can be detected by a number of laboratory tests such as radioimmunoassay or enzyme-linked immunosorbent assay (ELISA). Antibody to the surface antigen (anti-HBs) persists for many years. This antibody usually appears as the acute illness improves, providing protection against future HBV infections.

Hepatitis B Core Antigen (HBcAg). The HBV core protein can be identified only after the surface antigen has been stripped away using special techniques. Commercially available blood tests cannot detect HBcAg in blood, but antibody to the core antigen (anti-HBc) can be detected during acute illness. High levels of anti-HBc are present at the start of illness, and they gradually decrease over time in most people. In contrast, chronic carriers of HBV have high levels of anti-HBc in their blood that may persist throughout life.

E Antigen (HBeAg). The presence of e antigen indicates that a person infected with HBV is highly infectious. An HBsAg-positive pregnant woman whose blood contains e antigen is likely to transmit the virus to her newborn. By contrast, antibody to the e antigen (anti-HBe) may point to a lower degree of infectivity and a reduced likelihood of becoming a carrier. Laboratory blood tests can detect e antigen as well as anti-HBe.

Liver Function Tests. A number of blood tests can be performed to determine how well a person's liver is functioning, and these results can aid in diagnosing hepatitis B infection. High levels of the liver enzymes aspartate transferase (AST) and alanine transferase (ALT) are of particular importance. (These were formerly called SGOT and SGPT.)

Delta hepatitis. Until recently, delta hepatitis could be diagnosed only by liver biopsy in which a tiny piece of the liver is removed and examined. Scientists have developed a procedure to detect part of the genetic material of the virus in a patient's blood, which will allow easier, faster diagnosis. A blood test is also now available to detect antibody to delta antigen (a protein found inside the delta hepatitis virus).

Hepatitis C. A new test is now available to detect hepatitis C. The test identifies antibody to HCV, which is present in more than 50 percent of persons with acute hepatitis C and in almost all with chronic hepatitis.

Treatment

At present, there are no specific treatments for the acute symptoms of viral hepatitis. Doctors recommend bed rest, a healthy diet, and avoidance of alcoholic beverages to reduce stress on the liver.

A genetically engineered form of a naturally occurring protein, interferon alpha, is used to treat people with chronic hepatitis C. Studies supported by the National Institutes of Health (NIH) led to the approval of interferon alpha for the treatment of those with chronic HBV as well. The drug improves liver function in some people with hepatitis and diminishes symptoms, although it may cause side effects such as headache, fever, and other flu-like symptoms. Some patients do not respond to interferon alpha, and in others its beneficial effects lessen over time. Scientists are evaluating a number of experimental therapies that may be more effective and less toxic.

Possible Complications

Most patients with mild to severe acute hepatitis begin to feel better in 2 to 3 weeks and recover completely within 4 to 8 weeks. People with acute HBV infection who develop an HCV infection at the same time may be at particular risk for developing severe, life-threatening acute hepatitis.

Many chronic carriers remain symptom free or develop only a mild condition, chronic persistent hepatitis. However, a small percentage go on to develop the most serious complications of viral hepatitis: cirrhosis of the liver, liver cancer, and immune system disorders. Chronic carriers of HBV who become infected with HDV may develop severe acute hepatitis. They also have a high risk of becoming carriers of HDV.

Prevention

The most effective means of preventing viral hepatitis is to avoid contact with the blood, saliva, semen, or vaginal secretions of infected individuals. People who have acute or chronic viral hepatitis should:

Avoid sharing items that could infect others, such as razors or toothbrushes.

Protect sex partners from exposure to their semen, vaginal fluids, or blood. Properly used condoms may be effective in preventing sexual transmission.

There are several vaccines available to prevent hepatitis B. People at high risk of infection should consider vaccination: male homosexuals and heterosexuals with multiple partners, people who receive hemodialysis or blood products, household and sexual contacts of HBV carriers, and users of intravenous street drugs who share needles. Regulations now require health care and laboratory workers who handle blood and other body fluids to be vaccinated. People who have come into direct contact with the blood or body fluids of an HBV carrier may receive one or more injections of hepatitis B immune globulin, sometimes in combination with hepatitis B vaccine. Immune globulin offers temporary protection, while the vaccine provides a longer-lasting immunity.

In an effort to eliminate chronic carriers, the U.S. Centers for Disease Control recommends that all newborn babies be vaccinated. Other groups have recommended that pregnant women be screened for HBsAg as part of their routine prenatal care. If they are infected, their babies can be given hepatitis B immune globulin as well as vaccine immediately after birth.

No vaccines yet exist for HCV or HDV; however, HBV vaccine will prevent delta hepatitis as well.

Research

NIAID supported scientists are attacking hepatitis infection from several fronts. Work is under way to evaluate the potential of antiviral drugs to treat people already infected with HBV, HCV, and HDV. Vaccines and drugs are being tested in the woodchuck, an animal that develops a disease similar to HBV infection in humans. This animal also can be a chronic carrier of HDV, making it a valuable model for studying these viruses and helping scientists understand hepatitis infection.

In addition to testing their effectiveness, scientists are studying how to make antiviral drugs less toxic and how to deliver them to their appropriate targets in the body.

By studying the immune response to hepatitis viruses, scientists hope to identify the precise mechanisms that lead to either recovery or chronic disease. Knowledge is being gained from studies with transgenic mice (mice that carry human genes for HBV). By modifying viral genes and inoculating pregnant women, it may be possible to boost the immune response of babies to HBV. This approach could reduce a large number of chronic carriers and stem the spread of the disease to future generations.

HIV/AIDS

HIV/AIDS Diagnoses

At the end of 2003, an estimated 1,039,000 to 1,185,000 persons in the United States were living with HIV/AIDS, with 24-27% undiagnosed and unaware of their HIV infection.

AIDS Cases

In 2003, the estimated number of diagnoses of AIDS in the United States was 43,171. Adult and adolescent AIDS cases totaled 43,112 with 31,614 cases in males and 11,498 cases in females. Also in 2003, there were 59 AIDS cases estimated in children under age 13.

The cumulative estimated number of diagnoses of AIDS through 2003 in the United States is 929,985. Adult and adolescent AIDS cases total 920,566 with 749,887 cases in males and 170,679 cases in females. Through the same time period, 9,419 AIDS cases were estimated in children under age 13.

Deaths Due to AIDS

In 2003, the estimated number of deaths of persons with AIDS was 18,017, including 17,934 adults and adolescents, and 83 children under age 13

The cumulative estimated number of deaths of persons with AIDS through 2003 is 524,060, including 518,568 adults and adolescents, and 5,492 children under age 13.

AIDS Cases by Age

Of the estimated number of AIDS cases, person's age at time of diagnosis were distributed as follows:

Age	Estimated # of AIDS Cases in 2003	Cumulative Estimated # of AIDS Cases, Through 2003
Under 13:	59	9,419
Ages 13 to 14:	59	891
Ages 15 to 24:	1,991	37,599
Ages 25 to 34:	9,605	311,137
Ages 35 to 44:	17,633	365,432
Ages 45 to 54:	10,051	148,347
Ages 55 to 64:	2,888	43,451
Ages 65 or older:	886	13,711

AIDS Cases by Race/Ethnicity

Estimated diagnoses of AIDS, by race or ethnicity:

Race or Ethnicity	Estimated # of AIDS Cases in 2003	Cumulative Estimated # of AIDS Cases, Through 2003
White, not Hispanic	12,222	376,834
Black, not Hispanic	21,304	368,169
Hispanic	8,757	172,993
Asian/Pacific Islander	497	7,166
American Indian/Alaska Native	196	3,026

AIDS Cases by Exposure Category

Following is the distribution of the estimated number of diagnoses of AIDS among adults and adolescents by exposure category. A breakdown by sex is provided where appropriate.

Exposure Category	Estimated # of AIDS Cases, in 2003		
	Male	Female	Total
Male-to-male sexual contact	17,969	-	17,969
Injection Drug Use	6,353	3,096	9,449
Male-to-male sexual contact and injection drug use	1,877	-	1,877
Heterosexual contact	5,133	8,127	13,260
Other*	281	276	557

Exposure Category	Estimated # of AIDS Cases, Through 2003		
	Male	Female	Total
Male-to-male sexual contact	440,887	-	440,887
Injection Drug Use	175,988	70,558	246,546
Male-to-male sexual contact and injection drug use	62,418	-	62,418
Heterosexual contact	56,403	93,586	149,989
Other*	14,191	6,535	20,726

* Includes hemophilia, blood transfusion, perinatal, and risk not reported or not
  identified.

The distribution of the estimated number of diagnoses of AIDS, among children* by exposure categories follows:

Exposure Category	Estimated # of AIDS Cases in 2003	Cumulative Estimated # of AIDS Cases Through 2003
Perinatal	58	8,749
Other**	1	670

* The term "children" refers to persons under age 13 at the time of diagnosis.

** Includes hemophilia, blood transfusion, and risk not reported or not identified.

Top 10 AIDS Cases by State/Territory

The 10 states or territories reporting the highest number of AIDS cases are as follows:

# of AIDS Cases in 2003	State/Territory
6,684	New York
5,903	California
4,666	Florida
3,379	Texas
1,907	Georgia
1,895	Pennsylvania
1,730	Illinois
1.570	Maryland
1,516	New Jersey
1,083	North Carolina

# of Cumulative AIDS Cases Through 2003	State/Territory
162,446	New York
133,292	California
94,725	Florida
62,983	Texas
46,703	New Jersey
30,139	Illinois
29,988	Pennsylvania
28,301	Puerto Rico
27,915	Georgia
26,918	Maryland

In 2003, 32,048 cases of HIV/AIDS were reported from the 33 areas (32 states and the US Virgin Islands) with long-term, confidential name-based HIV reporting. When all 50 states are considered, CDC estimates that approximately 40,000 persons become infected with HIV each year.

By Exposure

In 2003, men who have sex with men (MSM) represented the largest proportion of HIV/AIDS diagnoses, followed by adults and adolescents infected through heterosexual contact.

Exposure categories of adults and adolescents who received a diagnosis of HIV/AIDS, 2003

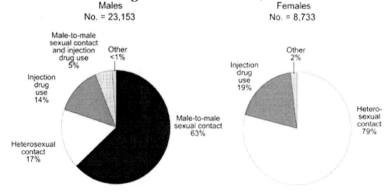

No. = 31,886

Note. Based on data from 33 areas with long-term, confidential name-based HIV reporting.

HIV/AIDS includes all persons with a diagnosis of HIV infection.

26

By Sex—In 2003, almost three quarters of HIV/AIDS diagnoses were made for male adolescents and adults.

Sex of adults and adolescents who received a diagnosis of HIV/AIDS, 2003

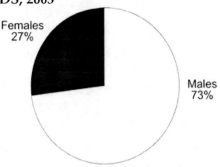

No. = 31,886

Note. Based on data from 33 areas with long-term, confidential name-based HIV reporting.

By Race/Ethnicity—Persons of minority races and ethnicities are disproportionately affected by HIV/AIDS. In 2003, African Americans, who make up approximately 12% of the US population, accounted for half of the HIV/AIDS cases diagnosed.

Race/ethnicity of persons (including children) who received a diagnosis of HIV/AIDS, 2003

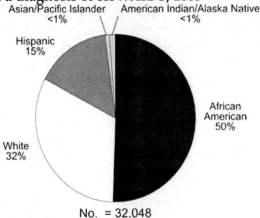

No. = 32,048

Note. Based on data from 33 areas with long-term, confidential name-based HIV reporting. Includes persons of unknown race or multiple races.

Trends in AIDS Diagnoses and Deaths

During the mid-to-late 1990s, advances in treatment slowed the progression of HIV infection to AIDS and led to dramatic decreases in AIDS deaths. Although the decrease in AIDS deaths continues (3% decrease from 1999 through 2003), the number of AIDS diagnoses increased an estimated 4% during that period.

Better treatments have also led to an increasing number of persons in the United States who are living with AIDS. From the end of 1999 through the end of 2003, the number of persons in the United States who were living with AIDS increased from 311,205 to 405,926—an increase of 30%.

Estimated AIDS diagnoses, deaths, and persons living with AIDS 1998–2002

	1999	2000	2001	2002	2003	Cumulative Through 2003
Estimated AIDS diagnoses	41,356	41,267	40,833	41,289	43,171	929,985
Estimated AIDS deaths	18,491	17,741	18,524	17,557	18,017	524,060
Estimated Persons living with AIDS	311,205	334,731	357,040	380,771	405,926	NA

NA, not applicable (the category Estimated persons living with AIDS is cumulative)

References

Glynn M, Rhodes P. Estimated HIV prevalence in the United States at the end of 2003. National HIV Prevention Conference; June 2005; Atlanta. Abstract 595.

CDC. HIV/AIDS Surveillance Report, 2003 (Vol. 15). Atlanta: US Department of Health and Human Services, CDC; 2004:1–46..

Other STDs

Chancroid

Since 1987, reported cases of chancroid had declined steadily until 2001 when 38 cases were reported (Figure 38, Table 1). In 2004, 30 cases of chancroid were reported in the United States. Only 16 states and one outlying area reported one or more cases of chancroid in 2004 (Table 45). Although the overall decline in reported chancroid cases most likely reflects a decline in the incidence of this disease, these data should be interpreted with caution in view of the fact that Haemophilus ducreyi, the causative organism of chancroid, is difficult to culture and, as a result, this condition may be substantially under diagnosed.[1, 2]

Chancroid - Reported cases: United States, 1981-2004

Cases (in thousands)

Human Papillomavirus

Sentinel surveillance for cervical infection with high-risk human papillomavirus (HR-HPV types 16, 18, 31, 33, 35, 39, 45, 51, 52, 56, 58, 59, 68) is being conducted in 29 STD, family planning and primary care clinics in six locations (Boston, MA; Baltimore, MD; New Orleans, LA; Denver, CO; Seattle, WA; and Los Angeles, CA) as part of an effort to estimate national burden of disease and inform prevention efforts in the U.S. Testing was performed using a commercially available test for HR-HPV testing (Digene Hybrid Capture 2, Gaithersburg, MD). Interim results from 2003-2004 document an overall HR-HPV prevalence of 22.5%. Prevalence in STD clinics was 28%, 24% in Family Planning clinics, and 16% in Primary Care clinics. Prevalence by age group was: 14-19 years 35%; 20-29 years 29%; 30-39 years 14%; 40-49 years 12%; and 50-65 years 6%.[3]

Lymphogranuloma Venereum

Lymphogranuloma venereum (LGV) is a systemic, sexually transmitted disease caused by a type of Chlamydia trachomatis. Prevalent in developing countries, LGV has been relatively rare in industrialized countries. However, beginning in late 2003 and continuing to the present time, outbreaks of LGV proctitis among men who have sex with men (MSM), the majority of whom were HIV infected, have been reported in Europe.[4, 5] There is no national surveillance for LGV in the United States. In 1995, LGV was removed from the list of nationally notifiable diseases. However, reporting is mandated in 24 states, and some of these states continue to report cases of LGV to the CDC. In 2004, 27 cases of LGV were reported to the CDC. Studies are underway to identify LGV throughout the United States through genotypic confirmation.6 Additional information can be found here.

Pelvic Inflammatory Disease

For data on Pelvic Inflammatory Disease (PID), see the Special Focus Profile on Women and Infants.

Other Sexually Transmitted Diseases

Case reporting data for genital herpes simplex virus (HSV), genital warts or other human papillomavirus infections, and trichomoniasis are not available. Trend data are limited to estimates of the office visits in physicians' office practices provided by the National Disease and Therapeutic Index (NDTI)

Genital herpes - Initial visits to physicians' offices: United States, 1966-2004

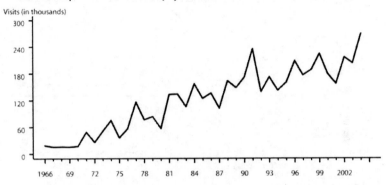

Genital warts - Initial visits to physicians' offices: United States, 1966-2004

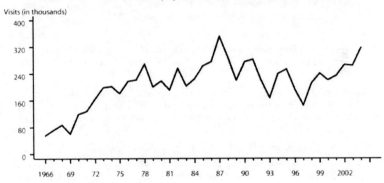

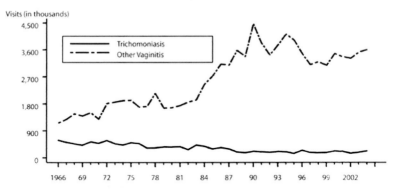

Trichomoniasis and other vaginal infections in women - Initial visits to physicians' offices: United States, 1966-2004

References:

1 Schulte JM, Martich FA, Schmid GP. Chancroid in the United States, 1981-1990: Evidence for underreporting of cases. MMWR 1992; 41(no. SS-3):57-61.

2 Mertz KJ, Trees D, Levine WC, et al. Etiology of genital ulcers and prevalence of human immunodeficiency virus coinfection in 10 US cities. J Infect Dis 1998;178:1795-8.

3 Datta SD, Koutsky L, Douglas J, et al. Sentinel surveillance for human papillo-mavirus among women in the United States, 2003-2004. Program and abstracts of the 16th Biennial Meeting of the International Society for Sexually Transmitted Diseases Research; July 10-13, 2005; Amsterdam, The Netherlands. Abstract MO-306.

4 Centers for Disease Control and Prevention. Lymphogranuloma venereum among men who have sex with men - Netherlands, 2003-2004. MMWR 2004; 53:985-988.

5 Nieuwenhuis RF, Ossewaarde JM, Götz HM, Dees J, Thio HB, Thomeer MG, et al. Resurgence of lymphogranuloma venereum in Western Europe: an outbreak of Chlamydia trachomatis serovar L2 proctitis in the Netherlands among men who have sex with men. Clin Infect Dis 2004;39:996-1003.

6 McLean C, Lindstrom H, Wendt A, et al. Lymphogranuloma venereum in the United States, November 2004 through March 2005. Program and abstracts of the 16th Biennial Meeting of the International Society for Sexually Transmitted Diseases Research; July 10-13, 2005; Amsterdam, The Netherlands. Poster MP-138.

Trends in STDs Special Focus Profiles

The Special Focus Profiles highlight trends and distribution of sexually transmitted diseases (STDs) in populations of particular interest for STD and HIV prevention programs in state and local health departments. These populations are most vulnerable to STDs and their consequences: women and infants, adolescents and young adults, minorities, men who have sex with men (MSM), and persons entering corrections facilities. The Special Focus Profiles refer to figures located in disease-specific sections in the National Profile and additional figures and tables (Figures A-GG and Tables AA-FF) that highlight specific points made in the text.

Women and Infants

Public Health Impact

Women and infants disproportionately bear the long term consequences of STDs. Women infected with *Neisseria gonorrhoeae* or *Chlamydia trachomatis* can develop pelvic inflammatory disease (PID), which, in turn, may lead to reproductive system morbidity such as ectopic pregnancy and tubal factor infertility. If not adequately treated, 20% to 40% of women infected with chlamydia[1] and 10% to 40% of women infected with gonorrhea[2] may develop PID. Among women with PID, tubal scarring will cause involuntary infertility in 20%, ectopic pregnancy in 9%, and chronic pelvic pain in 18%.[3] Approximately 70% of chlamydia infections and 50% of gonococcal [4-6] infections in women are asymptomatic. These infections are detected primarily through screening programs. The vague symptoms associated with chlamydial and gonococcal PID cause 85% of women to delay seeking medical care, thereby increasing the risk of infertility and ectopic pregnancy.[7] Data from a randomized controlled trial of chlamydia screening in a managed care setting suggest that such screening programs can reduce the incidence of PID by as much as 60%.[8]

Gonorrhea and chlamydia can also result in adverse outcomes of pregnancy, including neonatal ophthalmia and, in the case of chlamydia, neonatal pneumonia. Although topical prophylaxis of infants at delivery is effective for prevention of ophthalmia neonatorum, prevention of neonatal pneumonia requires prenatal detection and treatment.

Human papillomavirus (HPV) infections are highly prevalent, especially among young sexually active women. While the great majority of HPV infections in women resolve within one year, they are a major concern because persistent infection with specific types (e.g., types 16, 18, 31, 33, 35, and 45), are causally related to cervical cancer; these types also cause Pap smear abnormalities. Other types (e.g., types 6 and 11) cause genital warts, low grade Pap smear abnormalities and, rarely, recurrent respiratory papillomatosis in infants born to infected mothers.[9]

Genital infections with herpes simplex virus are extremely common, may cause painful outbreaks, and may have serious consequences for pregnant women including potentially fatal neonatal infections.[10]

When a woman has a syphilis infection during pregnancy, she may transmit the infection to the fetus in utero. This may result in fetal death or an infant born with physical and mental developmental disabilities. Most cases of congenital syphilis are easily preventable if women are screened for syphilis and treated early during prenatal care.[11]

Observations

Chlamydia and Gonorrhea

- Between 2003 and 2004, the rate of chlamydia infections in women increased from 463.6 to 485.0 per 100,000 females (Figure 5, Table 4). Chlamydia rates exceed gonorrhea rates among women in all states (Figures A and B, Tables 4 and 14).

- In 2004, the median state-specific chlamydia test positivity among 15- to 24-year-old women screened in selected prenatal clinics in 25 states, Puerto Rico, and the Virgin Islands was 6.8% (range 3.1% to 17.6%) (Figure E).

- In 2004, the median state-specific chlamydia test positivity among 15- to 24-year-old women who were screened during visits to selected family planning clinics in all states and outlying areas was 6.3% (range 3.2% to 16.3%) (Figure 7).

- Gonorrhea rates among women were higher than the overall HP 2010 target of 19.0 cases per 100,000 population[12] in 44 states and two outlying areas in 2004 (Figure B, Table 14).

- Like chlamydia, gonorrhea is often asymptomatic in women and can only be identified through screening. Large-scale screening programs for gonorrhea in women began in the 1970s. After an initial increase in cases detected through screening, gonorrhea rates for both women and men declined steadily throughout the 1980s and early 1990s (Figure 14 and Tables 14-15). The gonorrhea rate for women in 2004 (116.5 per 100,000 females) showed a slight decline since 2000. Although the gonorrhea rate in men has been historically higher than the rate in women, the gonorrhea rate among women has been higher than the rate among men for four consecutive years (Figure 14 and Tables 14-15).

- In 2004, the median state-specific gonorrhea test positivity among 15- to 24-year-old women screened in selected prenatal clinics in 19 states, Puerto Rico, and the Virgin Islands was 0.9% (range 0% to 3.5%) (Figure F).

35

- In 2004, the median state-specific gonorrhea test positivity among 15- to 24-year-old women screened in selected family planning clinics in 38 states, Puerto Rico, the District of Columbia, and the Virgin Islands was 1% (range 0.1%-4.2%).

Primary and Secondary Syphilis

- The HP2010 target for primary and secondary (P&S) syphilis is 0.2 case per 100,000 population. In 2004, 31 states, the District of Columbia, and two outlying areas had rates of P&S syphilis for women that were greater than 0.2 case per 100,000 population (Tables 27 and 31).

Congenital Syphilis

- The HP2010 target for congenital syphilis is 1.0 case per 100,000 live births. In 2004, 31 states and Puerto Rico had rates higher than this target (Figure 37, Tables 40, 41, 42).

- The number of congenital syphilis cases closely follows the trend of P&S syphilis among women (Figure 36). Peaks in congenital syphilis usually occur one year after peaks in P&S syphilis among women. The congenital syphilis rate peaked in 1991 at 107.3 cases per 100,000 live births, and declined by 92% to 8.8 cases per 100,000 live births in 2004 (Figure 36, Table 39). The rate of P&S syphilis among women declined 95.4% (from 17.3 to 0.8 cases per 100,000 females) during 1990-2004 (Figure 30).

- The 2004 rate of congenital syphilis for the United States is currently 9 times higher than the HP2010 target of 1.0 case per 100,000 live births. This target is many times greater than the rate of congenital syphilis of most industrialized countries where syphilis and congenital syphilis have nearly been eliminated.

- While most cases of congenital syphilis occur among infants whose mothers have had some prenatal care, late or limited prenatal care has been associated with congenital syphilis. Failure of health care providers to adhere to maternal syphilis screening recommendations also contributes to the occurrence of congenital syphilis.[13]

Pelvic Inflammatory Disease

- Accurate estimates of pelvic inflammatory disease (PID) and tubal factor infertility resulting from gonococcal and chlamydia infections are difficult to obtain. Definitive diagnosis of these conditions can be complex.

- Hospitalizations for PID have declined steadily throughout the 1980s and early 1990s, but have remained relatively constant between 1995 and 2003 (Figure H). A greater proportion of women diagnosed with PID in the 1990s have been treated in outpatient instead of inpatient settings when compared to women diagnosed with PID in the 1980s.[14]

- The reported number of initial visits to physicians' offices for PID through the National Disease and Therapeutic Index (NDTI) has generally declined from 1993 through 2004 (Figure I and Table 47).

- In 2002, an estimated 189,662 cases of PID were diagnosed in emergency departments among women 15 to 44 years of age. In 2003 this estimate decreased to 168,837 (National Hospital Ambulatory Medical Care Survey, NCHS). As of the date of publication of this report, 2004 data are not available.

Ectopic Pregnancy

- Evidence suggests that health care practices associated with ectopic pregnancy changed in the late 1980s and early 1990s. Before that time, treatment of ectopic pregnancy usually required admission to a hospital. Hospitalization statistics were therefore useful for monitoring trends in ectopic pregnancy. Beginning in 1989, hospitalizations for ectopic pregnancy have generally declined over time. Data suggest that nearly half of all ectopic pregnancies are treated on an outpatient basis.[15]

References

[1] Stamm WE, Guinan ME, Johnson C. Effect of treatment regimens for *Neisseria gonorrhoeae* on simultaneous infections with *Chlamydia trachomatis*. N Engl J Med 1984;310:545-9.

[2] Platt R, Rice PA, McCormack WM. Risk of acquiring gonorrhea and prevalence of abnormal adnexal findings among women recently exposed to gonorrhea. *JAMA* 1983;250:3205-9.

[3] Westrom L, Joesoef R, Reynolds G, et al. Pelvic inflammatory disease and fertility: a cohort study of 1,844 women with laparoscopically verified disease and 657 control women with normal laparoscopy. *Sexually Transmitted Diseases* 1992;9:185-92.

[4] Hook EW III, Handsfield HH. Gonococcal infections in the adult. In: Holmes KK, Mardh PA, Sparling PF, et al, eds. *Sexually Transmitted Diseases*, 2nd edition. New York City: McGraw-Hill, Inc, 1990:149-65.

[5] Stamm WE, Holmes KK. *Chlamydia trachomatis* infections in the adult. In: Holmes KK, Mardh PA, Sparling PF, et al, eds. *Sexually Transmitted Diseases*, 2nd edition. New York City: McGraw-Hill, Inc, 1990:181-93.

[6] Zimmerman HL, Potterat JJ, Dukes RL, et al. Epidemiologic differences between chlamydia and gonorrhea. *Am J Public Health* 1990;80:1338-42.

[7] Hillis SD, Joesoef R, Marchbanks PA, et al. Delayed care of pelvic inflammatory disease as a risk factor for impaired fertility. *Am J Obstet Gynecol* 1993;168:1503-9.

[8] Scholes D, Stergachis A, Heidrich FE, Andrilla H, Holmes KK, Stamm WE. Prevention of pelvic inflammatory disease by screening for cervical chlamydial infection. *N Engl J Med* 1996;34(21):1362-6.

[9] Division of STD Prevention. *Prevention of Genital HPV Infection and Sequelae: Report of an External Consultants' Meeting*. National Center for HIV, STD, and TB Prevention, Centers for Disease Control and Prevention, Atlanta, December 1999.

[10] Handsfield HH, Stone KM, Wasserheit JN. Prevention agenda for genital herpes. *Sexually Transmitted Diseases* 1999;26:228-231.

[11] Centers for Disease Control. Guidelines for prevention and control of congenital syphilis. *MMWR* 1988;37(No.S-1).

[12] U.S. Department of Health and Human Services. *Healthy People 2010*. 2nd ed. With Understanding and Improving Health and Objectives for Improving Health. 2 vols. Washington, DC: U.S. Government Printing Office, November 2000.

[13] Centers for Disease Control and Prevention. Congenital syphilis - United States, 2002. *MMWR* 2004;53:716-9.

[14] Rolfs RT, Galaid EI, Zaidi AA. Pelvic inflammatory disease: trends in hospitalization and office visits, 1979 through 1988. *Am J Obstet Gynecol* 1992;166:983-90.

[15] Centers for Disease Control and Prevention. Ectopic pregnancy in the United States, 1990-1992. *MMWR* 1995;44:46-8.

Adolescents and Young Adults

Public Health Impact

Compared to older adults, sexually active adolescents (10- to 19-year-olds) and young adults (20- to 24-year-olds) are at higher risk for acquiring STDs for a combination of behavioral, biological, and cultural reasons. For some STDs, for example, *Chlamydia trachomatis*, adolescent women may have a physiologically increased susceptibility to infection due to increased cervical ectopy. The higher prevalence of STDs among adolescents also reflects multiple barriers to quality STD prevention services, including lack of insurance or other ability to pay, lack of transportation, discomfort with facilities and services designed for adults, and concerns about confidentiality. Recent estimates suggest that while representing 25% of the ever sexually active population, 15- to 24-year olds acquire nearly one-half of all new STDs.[1]

Observations

Chlamydia and Gonorrhea

- Numerous prevalence studies in various clinic populations have shown that sexually active adolescents have high rates of chlamydia infection.[2-4] The Re-

39

gional Infertility Prevention Projects that routinely perform large scale screening for detecting chlamydia infections among women attending family planning clinics demonstrate that younger women consistently have higher positivity than older women, even when overall prevalence declines. An example is the Region X Chlamydia Project, which has screened women in family planning clinics since 1988 (Figure K).

- After adjusting trends in chlamydia positivity to account for changes in laboratory test methods and associated increases in test sensitivity (see Appendix), in 15- to 19-year-old women chlamydia test positivity decreased in 2 of 10 HHS regions from 2003 through 2004, increased in 7 regions, and remained the same in 1 region (Figure J).

- As in previous years, 15- to 19-year-old women had the highest rates of gonorrhea compared to women in all other age categories (Figure 17 and Table 20). Women aged 20-24 had the highest rates of primary and secondary syphilis in 2004, while among men, 35- to 39-year-olds had the highest rates of primary and secondary syphilis (Figure 34 and Table 33). Among men, 20- to 24-year-olds had the highest rate of gonorrhea (Figure 18 and Table 20).

- In 15- to 19-year-old women, the 2004 gonorrhea rate of 610.9 cases per 100,000 females was a 12.7% decrease from the 2000 rate of 699.5. Among young women in the 20- to 24-year-old group, the rate of gonorrhea in 2004 decreased 8.4% from 621.0 in 2000 to 569.1 in 2004 (Figure 17, Table 20).

- Rates of gonorrhea among male adolescents decreased between the years 2000 and 2004 (Figure 18, Table 20). Among 15- to 19-year-old males, the gonorrhea rate declined by 21.1% from 320.6 in 2000 to 252.9 in 2004. Among 20- to 24-year-old males, the gonorrhea rate declined by 22.3% from 554.1 in 2000 to 430.6 in 2004.

Primary and Secondary Syphilis

- Syphilis rates in women are highest in the 20-24 year age group, 3.0 cases per 100,000 population. Rates among 15-19 year olds have decreased over time and remain low (Figure 34, Table 33).

- In men, increases have been observed in 20- to 24-year-olds (Figure 35), but rates among 15-19 year olds are low and remain relatively unchanged (Figure 35, Table 33).

National Job Training Program

- Since 1990, approximately 20,000 female National Job Training Program entrants have been screened each year for chlamydia. This program, administered by the National Job Training Program at more than 100 sites throughout the country, is a job training program for economically-disadvantaged youth aged 16-24 years-old.

- Chlamydia infection is widespread geographically and highly prevalent among economically-disadvantaged young women in the National Job Training Program.[4] Among women entering the program from 38 states and Puerto Rico in 2004, based on their place of residence before program entry, the median state-specific chlamydia prevalence was 9.7% (range 4.4% to 17.3%) (Figure L). Among men entering the program from 46 states, the District of Columbia, and Puerto Rico in 2004, the median state-specific chlamydia prevalence was 7.3% (range 0.8% to 13%) (Figure M).

41

- Data from National Job Training Program centers that submit gonorrhea specimens from female students aged 16-24 years to a national contract laboratory indicates a high prevalence of gonococcal infection in this population. Specimens from at least 100 students from each of 33 states were tested by the contract laboratory; the median state-specific gonorrhea prevalence was 2.4% (range 0% to 6.4%) in 2004 (Figure N). Among men entering the program from 8 states in 2004, the median state-specific gonorrhea prevalence was 3.7% (range 1% to 5.5%) (Figure O).

Corrections Facilities

- Among adolescent women attending juvenile corrections facilities, data from the Corrections STD Prevalence Monitoring Project identified a median chlamydia positivity of 14% (range 2.4% to 26.5%) (Table AA) and a median gonorrhea positivity of 4.5% (range 0% to 16.6%) (Table CC). See Special Focus Profiles (STDs in Persons Entering Corrections Facilities).

[1] Weinstock, H, Berman, S, Cates, W, Jr. Sexually Transmitted Diseases among American Youth: Incidence and Prevalence Estimates, 2000. *Perspect Sex Reprod Health*, 2004:36(1):6-10.

[2] Centers for Disease Control and Prevention. Recommendations for the prevention and management of *Chlamydia trachomatis* infections, 1993. *MMWR* 1993;42(No. RR-12).

[3] Lossick J, DeLisle S, Fine D, Mosure DJ, Lee V, Smith C. Regional program for widespread screening for *Chlamydia trachomatis* in family planning clinics. In: Bowie WR, Caldwell HD, Jones RP, et al., eds. Chlamydial Infections: Proceedings of the Seventh International Symposium of Human Chlamydial Infections, Cambridge, *Cambridge University Press* 1990, pp. 575-9.

[4] Mertz KJ, Ransom RL, St. Louis ME, Groseclose SL, Hadgu A, Levine WC, Hayman C. Decline in the prevalence of genital chlamydia infection in young women entering a National Job Training Program, 1990-1997. *Am J Pub Health* 2001;91(8):1287-1290.

Racial and Ethnic Minorities

Public Health Impact

Surveillance data show higher rates of reported STDs among some minority racial or ethnic groups when compared with rates among whites. Race and ethnicity in the United States are risk markers that correlate with other more fundamental determinants of health status such as poverty, access to quality health care, health care seeking behavior, illicit drug use, and living in communities with high prevalence of STDs. Acknowledging the disparity in STD rates by race or ethnicity is one of the first steps in empowering affected communities to organize and focus on this problem.

Surveillance data are based on cases of STDs reported to state and local health departments (see Appendix). In many areas, reporting from public sources, (for example, STD clinics) is more complete than reporting from private sources. Since minority populations may utilize public clinics more than whites, differences in rates between minorities and whites may be increased by this reporting bias.

In 2004, 23.3% of reports on gonorrhea cases were missing information on race or ethnicity, and 29.3% of reports on chlamydia cases were missing race or ethnicity (Table A1). To adjust for missing data, cases in which information is unknown are redistributed according to the distribution of cases in which race or ethnicity is known. This process may exacerbate the reporting bias.

Observations

Chlamydia

- Although chlamydia in women is a widely distributed STD among all racial and ethnic groups, trends in positivity in women screened in HHS Region X show consistently higher chlamydia positivity among minorities (Figure P).

43

- In 2004, the rate of chlamydia among African-American females in the United States was more than 7 times higher than the rate among white females (1,722.3 and 226.6 per 100,000, respectively) (Table 11B). The chlamydia rate among African-American males was more than 11 times higher than that among white males (645.2 and 57.3 per 100,000 population, respectively).

Gonorrhea

- In 2004, 69.6% of the total number of cases of gonorrhea reported to CDC occurred among African-Americans (Table 21A). In 2004, the rate of gonorrhea among African-Americans was 629.6 cases per 100,000 population, among American Indian/Alaska Natives the rate was 117.7, and among Hispanics the rate was 71.3. These rates are 19, 4, and 2 times higher, respectively, than the rate among whites in 2004 of 33.3 cases per 100,000 population. The rate of gonorrhea among Asian/Pacific Islanders in 2004 was 21.4 cases per 100,000 population (Figure 15, Table 21B).

- From 2000 through 2004, gonorrhea rates among African-Americans declined by 19.1% (778.1 and 629.6 cases per 100,000 population, respectively). During the same period, gonorrhea rates increased by 19.8% among whites, 19.4% among American Indian/Alaska Natives, and 3.8% among Hispanics, and decreased by 19.9% among Asian/Pacific Islanders (Table 21B).

- Gonorrhea rates in 2004 among African-American men were 26 times higher than among white men. Gonorrhea rates in 2004 among African-American women were 15 times higher than among white women (Figure Q).

- Gonorrhea rates in 2004 were highest for African-Americans aged 15-24 years among all racial, ethnic, and age categories. In 2004, African-American women aged 15-19 years had a gonorrhea rate of 2,790.5 cases per 100,000 females. This rate was 14 times greater than the 2004 rate among white females of similar age (201.7). African-American men in the 15- to 19-year-old age category had a 2004 gonorrhea rate of 1,390.1 cases per 100,000 males, which was 37 times higher than the rate among 15- to 19-year-old white males of 37.9 per 100,000. Among 20- to 24-year-olds in 2004, the gonorrhea rate among African-Americans was 17 times greater than that among whites (2,487.2 and 149.0 cases per 100,000 population, respectively) (Table 21B).

- Although gonorrhea rates decreased for most age and race/ethnic groups during the 1980s, they did not decrease for African-American adolescents during this period; African-American 15- to 19-year-old females did not show a decrease in rates until 1991 (Figure R). Decreases among 15- to 19-year old African-American males did not begin until 1992 (Figure S). From 2000 to 2004, gonorrhea rates among 15- to 19-year-old African-American females and males decreased 19.7% and 25.5%, respectively.

Primary and Secondary Syphilis
- The syphilis epidemic in the late 1980s occurred primarily among heterosexual, minority populations.[1] During the 1990s, the rate of primary and secondary (P&S) syphilis declined among all racial and ethnic groups (Figure 31). During 2000-2004, the rate continued to decline among African-Americans, but the overall rate of P&S syphilis and rates among non-Hispanic whites, Hispanics, Asian/Pacific Is-

landers, and American Indian/Alaska Natives increased; increases in P&S syphilis occurred only among men and the most rapid rate of increase occurred among non-Hispanic white men during this time (Table 34B).

- Between 2003 and 2004, the rates of primary and secondary syphilis increased 11% in white men, 17% in African-American men and increased slightly (2%) among African-American women (Table 34B). Rates continued to increase among Hispanics, Asian/Pacific Islanders, and American Indian/Alaska Natives.

- In 2004, 41% of all cases of P&S syphilis reported to CDC occurred among African-Americans and 40% of all cases occurred among non-Hispanic whites (Table 34A). The 2004 rate for African-Americans was 6 times greater than the rate among non-Hispanic whites (Table 34B).

- In 2004, the incidence of P&S syphilis by sex among African-Americans was highest among women aged 20-24 years (13.4 cases per 100,000 population) and among men aged 25-29 (34.6 cases per 100,000 population) (Table 34B). In 2003, African-American men in the 35-39 age group had the highest rates.

- Between 2003 and 2004, P&S syphilis rates for African-Americans in every age group increased. (Table 34B).

- In 2004, 16% of all cases of P&S syphilis reported to CDC occurred among Hispanics (Table 34A). The rate of P&S syphilis among Hispanic men increased 12% (from 4.9 to 5.5 cases per 100,000 population) between 2003 and 2004. The rate among Hispanic women remained essentially unchanged (0.7 cases per 100,000 population). The rate among Hispanics in 2004 was 2 times greater than the rate among non-Hispanic whites.

- The incidence of P&S syphilis among Hispanics was highest among women aged 20-24 years (1.9 cases per 100,000 population) and among men aged 35-39 years (14.0 cases per 100,000 population) in 2004 (Table 34B).

Congenital Syphilis

- In 2004, the rate of congenital syphilis (based on the mother's race/ethnicity) was 26.7 cases per 100,000 live births among African-Americans and 16.2 cases per 100,000 live births among Hispanics. These rates are 16 and 10 times greater, respectively, than the 2004 rate among non-Hispanic whites (1.7 cases per 100,000 live births), respectively (Figure W, Table 44).

[1] Nakashima AK, Rolfs RT, Flock ML, Kilmarx P, Greenspan JR. Epidemiology of syphilis in the United States, 1941 through 1993. *Sexually Transmitted Diseases* 1996;23:16-23.

Men Who Have Sex with Men

Public Health Impact

Data from several U.S. cities and projects, including syphilis outbreak investigations and the Gonococcal Isolate Surveillance Project (GISP), suggest that an increasing number of men who have sex with men (MSM) are acquiring STDs.[1-5] Data also suggest that an increasing number of MSM are engaging in sexual behaviors that place them at risk for STDs and HIV infection.[6] Several factors may be contributing to this change, including the availability of highly active antiretroviral therapy (HAART) for HIV infection.[7] Because STDs and the behaviors associated with them increase the likelihood of acquiring and transmitting HIV infection,[8] the rise in STDs among MSM may be associated with an increase in HIV incidence among MSM.[9]

Observations

- Nationally notifiable STD surveillance data reported to CDC do not include information regarding sexual behaviors; therefore, national trends in STDs among MSM in the United States are not available. Data from enhanced surveillance projects are presented in this section to provide information regarding STDs in MSM.

Monitoring Trends in Prevalence of STDs and HIV Risk Behaviors among Men Who Have Sex with Men (MSM Prevalence Monitoring Project)

- From 1999 through 2004, nine U.S. cities participating in the MSM Prevalence Monitoring Project submitted syphilis, gonorrhea, chlamydia, and HIV test data to CDC from 81,923 MSM visits to STD clinics; data from 68,917 MSM visits were submitted from six public STD clinics (Denver, Long Beach, New York City, Philadelphia, San Francisco, and Seattle) and 13,006 MSM visits were submitted from three STD clinics in community-based, gay men's health clinics (Chicago, the District of Columbia, and Houston). In 2004, eight U.S. cities submitted information from 18,186 MSM STD clinic visits.

- In 2004, Fenway Community Health (Boston), a community-based, gay men's primary care clinic, also participating in the MSM Prevalence Monitoring Project, submitted syphilis, gonorrhea, and chlamydia test data to CDC from 22,237 primary care visits by men.

- The MSM Prevalence Monitoring Project includes data from culture and non-culture tests collected during routine care and reflects testing practices at participating clinics. City-specific medians and ranges were calculated for the proportion of tests done and STD and HIV test positivity.

Syphilis, STD Clinics, 1999-2004

- In 2004, 85% (range: 63-91%) of MSM visiting participating STD clinics had a nontreponemal serologic test for syphilis (STS) [RPR or VDRL] performed compared with 69% (range: 54-93%) in 1999.

- Overall, median syphilis seroreactivity among MSM tested increased from 4% (range: 4-13%) in 1999 to 10% (range: 6-4%) in 2004 (Figure X).

Gonorrhea, STD Clinics, 1999-2004

- In 2004, overall median clinic gonorrhea positivity in MSM was 15% (range: 11-17%) at any anatomic site (Figure Y).

- In 2004, 80% (range: 57-95%) of MSM were tested for urethral gonorrhea, 34% (range: 3-65%) were tested for rectal gonorrhea, and 50% (range: 5-92%) were tested for pharyngeal gonorrhea.

- In 2004, median clinic urethral gonorrhea positivity in MSM was 11% (range: 7-13%), median rectal gonorrhea positivity was 8% (range: 3-19%), and median pharyngeal gonorrhea positivity was 5% (range: 3-14%).

- In 2004, by race/ethnicity, urethral gonorrhea positivity was 11% (range: 8-12%) in whites, 16% (range: 9-24%) in African-Americans, and 9% (range: 3-10%) in Hispanics. Rectal gonorrhea positivity was 7% (range: 4-12%) in whites, 6% (range: 2-8%) in African-Americans, and 5% (range: 3-8%) in Hispanics. Pharyngeal gonorrhea positivity was 6% (range: 3-14%) in whites, 7% (range: 1-10%) in African-Americans, and 4% (range: 2-10%) in Hispanics (Figure Z).

- In 2004, by HIV status, urethral gonorrhea positivity was 17% (range: 12-25%) in HIV-positive MSM and 10% (range 6-12%) in MSM who were HIV-negative or of unknown HIV status; rectal gonorrhea positivity was 10% (range: 4-12%) in HIV-positive MSM and 7% (range: 3-9%) in MSM who were HIV-negative or of unknown HIV status; pharyngeal gonorrhea positivity was 5% (range: 3-10%) in HIV-positive MSM and 5% (range: 3-13%) in MSM who were HIV-negative or of unknown HIV status (Figure AA).

HIV Infection, STD Clinics, 2004

- In 2004, a median of 59% (range: 30-81%) of MSM visiting STD clinics in the project and not previously known to be HIV-positive were tested for HIV; median HIV positivity was 4% (range: 2-6%). HIV positivity varied by race and ethnicity, but was higher in African-American and Hispanic MSM. HIV positivity was 3% (range: 2-4%) in whites, 7% (range 3-13%) in African-Americans, and 7% (range: 3-7%) in Hispanics (Figure Z).

- In 2004, median HIV prevalence among MSM, including persons previously known to be HIV-positive and persons testing HIV-positive at their current visit, was 11% (range 6-14%). HIV prevalence was 11% (range: 5-14%) in whites, 16% (range: 10-20%) in African-Americans, and 11% (range: 6-14%) in Hispanics (Figure AA).

Chlamydia, STD Clinics, 2004

- In 2004, a median of 82% (range: 57-95%) of MSM visiting participating STD clinics were tested for urethral chlamydia; median urethral chlamydia positivity was 6% (range: 5-8%). Urethral chlamydia was

5% (range: 2-8%) in whites; 9% (range: 8-11%) in African-Americans, and 6% (range: 3-14%) in Hispanics (Figure Z). Median positivity was 6% (range: 5-14%) in HIV-positive MSM and 6% (range: 5-7%) in MSM who were HIV-negative or of unknown HIV status (Figure AA).

STD Testing and Positivity, Community-based, Gay Men's Primary Care Clinic, 2004

- In 2004, among men with a nontreponemal serologic test for syphilis in a gay men's primary care clinic, 5% had a reactive syphilis test result and 31% of men with reactive syphilis serologies were identified as new syphilis cases. Among men tested for gonorrhea, urethral positivity was 9%, rectal positivity was 7%, and pharyngeal positivity was 2%. Among men tested for urethral chlamydia, positivity was 5%.

Nationally Reported Syphilis Surveillance Data

- Primary and secondary (P&S) syphilis increased in the United States during 2000-2004. Between 2000 and 2004, there was a 90% increase in the number of P&S syphilis cases among men and a 49% decrease in the number of cases among women (Tables 27 and 28). Trends in the syphilis male-to-female rate ratio, which are assumed to reflect syphilis trends among MSM, have been increasing in the United States during recent years (Figure 32). In 2004, the rate of reported P&S syphilis among men (4.7 cases per 100,000 males) was 6 times greater than the rate among women (0.8 cases per 100,000 females) (Figure T). The overall male-to-female syphilis rate ratio has risen steadily since 2000 when it was 1.5 (Figure 32). The increase in the male-to-female rate ratio occurred among all racial and ethnic groups between 2000 and 2004. Additional information on syphilis can be found in the Syphilis section.

Gonococcal Isolate Surveillance Project (GISP)

- The Gonococcal Isolate Surveillance Project (GISP), a collaborative project among selected STD clinics, was established in 1986 to monitor trends in antimicrobial susceptibilities of strains of *Neisseria gonorrhoeae* in the United States.[10]

- GISP also reports the percentage of *Neisseria gonorrhoeae* isolates obtained from MSM. Overall, the proportion of isolates coming from MSM in GISP clinics increased from 4% in 1988 to 20% in 2004, with most of the increase occurring after 1993 (Figure BB). Additional information on GISP may be found in the Gonorrhea section.

- The proportion of isolates coming from MSM varies geographically with the largest percentage from the west coast (Figure CC).

- Due to increases in the proportion of isolates from MSM that are fluoroquinolone-resistant (Figure 23), in 2004 CDC recommended that fluoroquinolones no longer be used to treat gonorrhea among MSM.[11]

[1] Centers for Disease Control and Prevention. Gonorrhea among men who have sex with men - selected sexually transmitted disease clinics, 1993-1996. *MMWR* 1997;46:889-92.

[2] Centers for Disease Control and Prevention. Resurgent bacterial sexually transmitted disease among men who have sex with men - King County, Washington, 1997-1999. *MMWR* 1999;48:773-7.

[3] Centers for Disease Control and Prevention. Outbreak of syphilis among men who have sex with men -Southern California, 2000. *MMWR* 2001;50:117-20.

[4] Fox KK, del Rio C, Holmes K, et. al. Gonorrhea in the HIV era: A reversal in trends among men who have sex with men. *Am J Public Health* 2001;91:959-964.

[5] Centers for Disease Control and Prevention. Primary and secondary syphilis among men who have sex with men - New York City, 2001. *MMWR* 2002;51:853-6.

[6] Stall R, Hays R, Waldo C, Ekstrand M, McFarland W. The gay '90s: a review of research in the 1990s on sexual behavior and HIV risk among men who have sex with men. *AIDS* 2000;14:S1-S14.

[7] Scheer S, Chu PL, Klausner JD, Katz MH, Schwarcz SK. Effect of highly active antiretroviral therapy on diagnoses of sexually transmitted diseases in people with AIDS. *Lancet* 2001;357:432-5.

[8] Fleming DT, Wasserheit JN. From epidemiologic synergy to public health policy and practice: the contribution of other sexually transmitted diseases to sexual transmission of HIV infection. *Sex Transm Infect* 1999;75:3-17.

[9] Centers for Disease Control and Prevention. *HIV/AIDS Surveillance Report*, 2003, (Vol. 15). Atlanta: U.S. Department of Health and Human Services, Centers for Disease Control and Prevention; 2004.

[10] Centers for Disease Control and Prevention. *Sexually Transmitted Disease Surveillance 2004 Supplement: Gonococcal Isolate Surveillance Project (GISP) Annual Report 2004*. Atlanta, GA: U.S. Department of Health and Human Services (available first quarter 2006).

[11] Centers for Disease Control and Prevention. Increases in fluoroquinolone-resistant *Neisseria gonorrhoeae* among men who have sex with men - United States, 2003, and revised recommendations for gonorrhea treatment, 2004. *MMWR* 2004;53:335-338.

Persons Entering Corrections Facilities

Public Health Impact

Multiple studies and surveillance projects have demonstrated a high prevalence of STDs in persons entering jails and juvenile corrections facilities. [1-4] Screening for chlamydia, gonorrhea, and syphilis at intake offers an opportunity to identify infections, prevent complications, and reduce transmission in the general community. For example, one study has suggested that screening and treatment of women inmates for syphilis may result in reduction of syphilis in the general community.[5] Depending on locale, a substantial proportion of all early syphilis cases are reported from corrections facilities.[4] Collecting positivity data and analyzing trends in STD prevalence in the inmate population can provide a tool for monitoring trends in STD prevalence in the general community.[4]

Description of Population

- In 2004, STD screening data from corrections facilities were reported from 34 states for chlamydia, 29 states for gonorrhea, and 10 states for syphilis. These data were reported in response to CDC's request for data, as part of the Corrections STD Prevalence Monitoring Project and/or the Regional Infertility Prevention Project.

- The tables and figures shown in this section represent 103,595 chlamydia tests in men and 60,466 in women; 77,043 gonorrhea tests in men and 44,161 in women; and 235,017 syphilis tests in men and 56,200 in women entering corrections facilities during 2004.

Chlamydia

- In adolescent men entering 81 juvenile corrections facilities, the median chlamydia positivity was 5.8% (range 1% to 27.5%) (Table AA). In adolescent women entering 56 juvenile corrections facilities, the median chlamydia positivity was 14% (range 2.4% to 26.5%); positivity was greater than 10% in 42 of 56 facilities reporting data.

- In men entering juvenile corrections facilities, chlamydia positivity increased from 1.0% for those aged 12 years to 8.0 % for those aged 17 years (Figure DD). For those aged 17 years to 19 years, the rates were similar. In women entering juvenile corrections facilities, chlamydia positivity increased from 8.5% for those aged 12 years to 16.9% for those aged 15 years.

- In men entering 35 adult corrections facilities, the median chlamydia positivity was 10.2% (range 0.7% to 30%) (Table BB). In women entering 32 adult corrections facilities, the median positivity for chlamydia was 7.2% (range 1.2% to 22.7%).

54

- In men entering adult corrections facilities, chlamydia positivity decreased with age from 10.7% for those aged 18-19 years to 1.9% for those aged 35 to 65 years (Figure EE). Similar trends were also observed in adult women. Although overall chlamydia positivity in women entering adult correction facilities was significantly lower than in women entering juvenile corrections facilities, chlamydia positivity in women aged 18-19 years attending adult corrections facilities was higher than in women attending juvenile corrections facilities. Similar patterns were also observed for men aged 20 years entering adult corrections facilities compared to men entering juvenile corrections facilities.

Gonorrhea

- The median positivity for gonorrhea in adolescent men entering 49 juvenile corrections facilities was 0.8% (range 0% to 18.2%) (Table CC). The median positivity for gonorrhea in women entering 34 juvenile corrections facilities was 4.5% (range 0% to 16.6%); positivity was greater than 4% in 20 of 34 juvenile corrections facilities.

- In men entering juvenile corrections facilities, gonorrhea positivity increased from 0.2% for those aged 12 years to 1.4% for those aged 19 years (Figure FF). This trend was not observed in adolescent women.

- In men entering 27 adult corrections facilities, the median positivity was 2.6% (range 0% to 33.8%) (Table DD). In women entering 26 adult facilities, the median positivity for gonorrhea was 3.0% (range 0% to 8.4%).

- In women entering adult corrections facilities, gonorrhea positivity decreased with age from 9.5% for those aged 18-19 years to 4.2% for those aged 35 to 65 years (Figure GG). This trend was not observed in adult men. Women aged 18-19 years attending adult facilities had higher gonorrhea positivity than women attending juvenile detention facilities. This was also true for men.

Syphilis

- The median reactive syphilis serology was 0.5% (range 0% to 2.4%) in adolescent men entering 5 corrections facilities and 0.7% (range 0% to 5.1%) in adolescent women entering 5 juvenile corrections facilities (Table EE).

- In men at 24 adult corrections facilities, the median reactive syphilis serology was 2.7% (range 0.2% to 5.9%) (Table FF). In women entering 19 adult corrections facilities the median percentage of reactive syphilis tests by facility was 5.3% (range 0% to 19%).

References

[1] Heimberger TS. Chang HG. Birkhead GS. DiFerdinando GD. Greenberg AJ. Gunn R. Morse DL. High prevalence of syphilis detected through a jail screening program. A potential public health measure to address the syphilis epidemic. *Arch Intern Med* 1993;153:1799-1804.

[2] Centers for Disease Control and Prevention. Syphilis screening among women arrestees at the Cook County Jail - Chicago, 1996. *MMWR* 1998;47:432-3.

[3] Mertz KJ, Schwebke JR, Gaydos CA, Beideinger HA, Tulloch SD, Levine WC. Screening women in jails for chlamydial and gonococcal infection using urine tests: Feasibility, acceptability, prevalence and treatment rates. *Sexually Transmitted Diseases* 2002;29:271-276.

[4] Kahn R, Voigt R, Swint E, Weinstock H. Early syphilis in the United States identified in corrections facilities, 1999-2002. *Sexually Transmitted Diseases* 2004;31:360-364.

[5] Blank S, McDonnell DD, Rubin SR et al., New approaches to syphilis control. Finding opportunities for syphilis treatment and congenital syphilis prevention in a women's correctional setting. *Sexually Transmitted Diseases* 1997; 24:218-26.

Section II
Information in Depth

Chlamydia

Chlamydia is the most frequently reported bacterial sexually transmitted disease in the United States. In 2002, 834,555 chlamydial infections were reported to CDC from 50 states and the District of Columbia. Under-reporting is substantial because most people with chlamydia are not aware of their infections and do not seek testing. Also, testing is not often done if patients are treated for their symptoms. An estimated 2.8 million Americans are infected with chlamydia each year. Women are frequently re-infected if their sex partners are not treated.

Chlamydia is caused by the bacterium, Chlamydia trachomatis, which can damage a woman's reproductive organs. Even though symptoms of chlamydia are usually mild or absent, serious complications that cause irreversible damage, including infertility, can occur "silently" before a woman ever recognizes a problem. Chlamydia also can cause discharge from the penis of an infected man.

Chlamydia can be transmitted during vaginal, anal, or oral sex. Chlamydia can also be passed from an infected mother to her baby during vaginal childbirth.

Any sexually active person can be infected with chlamydia. The greater the number of sex partners, the greater the risk of infection. Because the cervix (opening to the uterus) of teenage girls and young women is not fully matured, they are at particularly high risk for infection if sexually active. Since chlamydia can be transmitted by oral or anal sex, men who have sex with men are also at risk for chlamydial infection.

Symptoms

Chlamydia is known as a "silent" disease because about three quarters of infected women and about half of infected men have no symptoms. If symptoms do occur, they usually appear within 1 to 3 weeks after exposure.

In women, the bacteria initially infect the cervix and the urethra (urine canal). Women who have symptoms might have an abnormal vaginal discharge or a burning sensation when urinating. When the infection spreads from the cervix to the fallopian tubes (tubes that carry eggs from the ovaries to the uterus), some women still have no signs or symptoms; others have lower abdominal pain, low back pain, nausea, fever, pain during intercourse, or bleeding between menstrual periods. Chlamydial infection of the cervix can spread to the rectum.

Men with signs or symptoms might have a discharge from their penis or a burning sensation when urinating. Men might also have burning and itching around the opening of the penis. Pain and swelling in the testicles are uncommon.

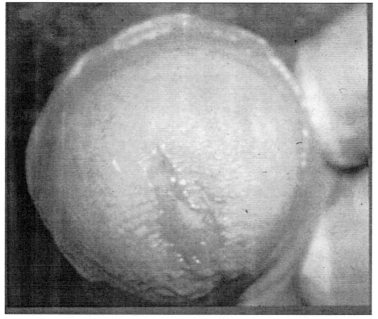

Men or women who have receptive anal intercourse may acquire chlamydial infection in the rectum, which can cause rectal pain, discharge, or bleeding. Chlamydia can also be found in the throats of women and men having oral sex with an infected partner.

If untreated, chlamydial infections can progress to serious reproductive and other health problems with both short-term and long-term consequences. Like the disease itself, the damage that chlamydia causes is often "silent."

In women, untreated infection can spread into the uterus or fallopian tubes and cause pelvic inflammatory disease (PID). This happens in up to 40 percent of women with untreated chlamydia. PID can cause permanent damage to the fallopian tubes, uterus, and surrounding tissues. The damage can lead to chronic pelvic pain, infertility, and potentially fatal ectopic pregnancy (pregnancy outside the uterus). Women infected with chlamydia are up to five times more likely to become infected with HIV, if exposed.

To help prevent the serious consequences of chlamydia, screening at least annually for chlamydia is recommended for all sexually active women age 25 years and younger. An annual screening test also is recommended for older women with risk factors for chlamydia (a new sex partner or multiple sex partners). All pregnant women should have a screening test for chlamydia.

Complications among men are rare. Infection sometimes spreads to the epididymis (a tube that carries sperm from the testis), causing pain, fever, and, rarely, sterility.

Rarely, genital chlamydial infection can cause arthritis that can be accompanied by skin lesions and inflammation of the eye and urethra (Reiter's syndrome).

Effects on Pregnancy

In pregnant women, there is some evidence that untreated chlamydial infections can lead to premature delivery. Babies who are born to infected mothers can get chlamydial infections in their eyes and respiratory tracts. Chlamydia is a leading cause of early infant pneumonia and conjunctivitis (pink eye) in newborns.

Diagnosis and Treatment

There are laboratory tests to diagnose chlamydia. Some can be performed on urine; other tests require that a specimen be collected from a site such as the penis or cervix.

Chlamydia can be easily treated and cured with antibiotics. A single dose of azithromycin or a week of doxycycline (twice daily) are the most commonly used treatments. HIV-positive persons with chlamydia should receive the same treatment as those who are HIV negative.

All sex partners should be evaluated, tested, and treated. Persons with chlamydia should abstain from sexual intercourse until they and their sex partners have completed treatment, otherwise re-infection is possible.

Women whose sex partners have not been appropriately treated are at high risk for re-infection. Having multiple infections increases a woman's risk of serious reproductive health complications, including infertility. Retesting should be considered for women, especially adolescents, three to four months after treatment. This is especially true if a woman does not know if her sex partner received treatment.

Prevention

The surest way to avoid transmission of sexually transmitted diseases is to abstain from sexual contact, or to be in a long-term mutually monogamous relationship with a partner who has been tested and is known to be uninfected.

Latex male condoms, when used consistently and correctly, can reduce the risk of transmission of chlamydia.

Chlamydia screening is recommended annually for all sexually active women 25 years of age and younger. An annual screening test also is recommended for older women with risk factors for chlamydia (a new sex partner or multiple sex partners). All pregnant women should have a screening test for chlamydia.

Any genital symptoms such as discharge or burning during urination or unusual sore or rash should be a signal to stop having sex and to consult a health care provider immediately. If a person has been treated for chlamydia (or any other STD), he or she should notify all recent sex partners so they can see a health care provider and be treated. This will reduce the risk that the sex partners will develop serious complications from chlamydia and will also reduce the person's risk of becoming re-infected. The person and all of his or her sex partners must avoid sex until they have completed their treatment for chlamydia.

Sources

Weinstock H, Berman S, Cates W. Sexually transmitted disease among American youth: Incidence and prevalence estimates, 2000. Perspectives on Sexual and Reproductive Health 2004; 36: 6-10.

Centers for Disease Control and Prevention. Sexually Transmitted Disease Surveillance, 2002. Atlanta, GA: U.S. Department of Health and Human Service, September 2003.

Stamm W E. Chlamydia trachomatis infections of the adult. In: K. Holmes, P. Sparling, P. Mardh et al (eds). Sexually Transmitted Diseases, 3rd edition. New York: McGraw-Hill, 1999, 407-422.

Centers for Disease Control and Prevention. Sexually Transmitted Diseases Treatment Guidelines 2002. MMWR 2002;51(no. RR-6).

Genital HPV

Approximately 20 million people are currently infected with HPV. At least 50 percent of sexually active men and women acquire genital HPV infection at some point in their lives. By age 50, at least 80 percent of women will have acquired genital HPV infection. About 6.2 million Americans get a new genital HPV infection each year.

Genital HPV infection is caused by human papillomavirus (HPV). Human papillomavirus is the name of a group of viruses that includes more than 100 different strains or types. More than 30 of these viruses are sexually transmitted, and they can infect the genital area of men and women including the skin of the penis, vulva (area outside the vagina), or anus, and the linings of the vagina, cervix, or rectum. Most people who become infected with HPV will not have any symptoms and will clear the infection on their own.

Some of these viruses are called "high-risk" types, and may cause abnormal Pap tests. They may also lead to cancer of the cervix, vulva, vagina, anus, or penis. Others are called "low-risk" types, and they may cause mild Pap test abnormalities or genital warts. Genital warts are single or multiple growths or bumps that appear in the genital area, and sometimes are cauliflower shaped.

The types of HPV that infect the genital area are spread primarily through genital contact. Most HPV infections have no signs or symptoms; therefore, most infected persons are unaware they are infected, yet they can transmit the virus to a sex partner. Rarely, a pregnant woman can pass HPV to her baby during vaginal delivery. A baby that is exposed to HPV very rarely develops warts in the throat or voice box.

Symptoms

Most people who have a genital HPV infection do not know they are infected. The virus lives in the skin or mucous membranes and usually causes no symptoms. Some people get visible genital warts, or have pre-cancerous changes in the cervix, vulva, anus, or penis. Very rarely, HPV infection results in anal or genital cancers.

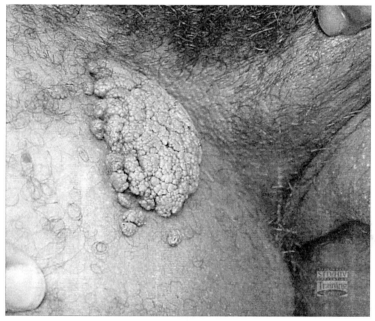

Genital Warts on the Thigh (source CDC STD101 slides)

Genital warts usually appear as soft, moist, pink, or flesh-colored swellings, usually in the genital area. They can be raised or flat, single or multiple, small or large, and sometimes cauliflower shaped. They can appear on the vulva, in or around the vagina or anus, on the cervix, and on the penis, scrotum, groin, or thigh. After sexual contact with an infected person, warts may appear within weeks or months, or not at all.

Genital warts are diagnosed by visual inspection. Visible genital warts can be removed by medications the patient applies, or by treatments performed by a health care provider. Some individuals choose to forego treatment to see if the warts will disappear on their own. No treatment regimen for genital warts is better than another and no one treatment regimen is ideal for all cases.

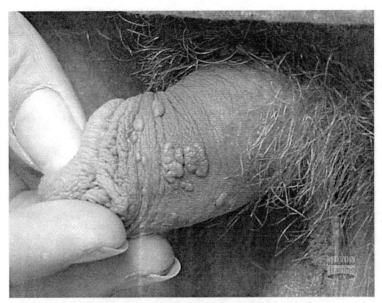

HPV Warts on the shaft of the penis (source CDC STD101 slides)

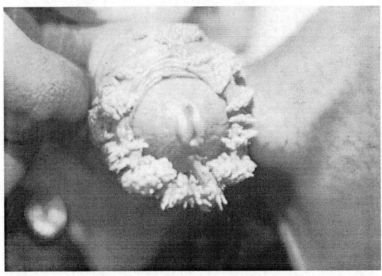

Condyloma acuminata, or *genital warts* on the penis (source CDC STD101 slides)

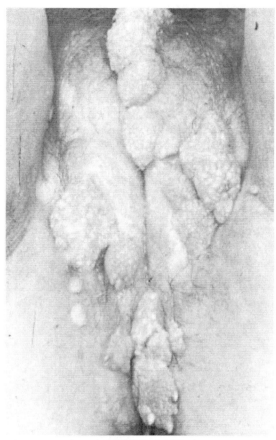

Genital warts in a woman (source CDC STD101 slides)

Diagnosis and treatment

Most women are diagnosed with HPV on the basis of abnormal Pap tests. A Pap test is the primary cancer-screening tool for cervical cancer or pre-cancerous changes in the cervix, many of which are related to HPV. Also, a specific test is available to detect HPV DNA in women. The test may be used in women with mild Pap test abnormalities, or in women >30 years of age at the time of Pap testing. The results of HPV DNA testing can help health care providers decide if further tests or treatment are necessary.

No HPV tests are available for men.

Genital HPV has no "cure"

There is no "cure" for HPV infection, although in most women the infection goes away on its own. The treatments provided are directed to the changes in the skin or mucous membrane caused by HPV infection, such as warts and pre-cancerous changes in the cervix.

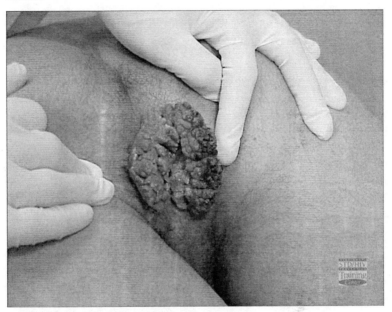

Perianal Wart (source CDC STD101 slides)

HPV and Cervical Cancer

All types of HPV can cause mild Pap test abnormalities which do not have serious consequences. Approximately 10 of the 30 identified genital HPV types can lead, in rare cases, to development of cervical cancer. Research has shown that for most women (90 percent), cervical HPV infection becomes undetectable within two years. Although only a small proportion of women have persistent infection, persistent infection with "high-risk" types of HPV is the main risk factor for cervical cancer.

A Pap test can detect pre-cancerous and cancerous cells on the cervix. Regular Pap testing and careful medical follow-up, with treatment if necessary, can help ensure that pre-cancerous changes in the cervix caused by HPV infection do not develop into life threatening cervical cancer. The Pap test used in U.S. cervical cancer screening programs is responsible for greatly reducing deaths from cervical cancer. For 2004, the American Cancer Society estimates that about 10,520 women will develop invasive cervical cancer and about 3,900 women will die from this disease. Most women who develop invasive cervical cancer have not had regular cervical cancer screening.

Prevention

The surest way to eliminate risk for genital HPV infection is to refrain from any genital contact with another individual.

For those who choose to be sexually active, a long-term, mutually monogamous relationship with an uninfected partner is the strategy most likely to prevent future genital HPV infections. However, it is difficult to determine whether a partner who has been sexually active in the past is currently infected.

For those choosing to be sexually active and who are not in long-term mutually monogamous relationships, reducing the number of sexual partners and choosing a partner less likely to be infected may reduce the risk of genital HPV infection. Partners less likely to be infected include those who have had no or few prior sex partners.

HPV infection can occur in both male and female genital areas that are covered or protected by a latex condom, as well as in areas that are not covered. While the effect of condoms in preventing HPV infection is unknown, condom use has been associated with a lower rate of cervical cancer, an HPV-associated disease.

Sources

Centers for Disease Control and Prevention. Sexually Transmitted Diseases Treatment Guidelines 2002. MMWR 2002;51(no. RR-6).

Ho GYF, Bierman R, Beardsley L, Chang CJ, Burk RD. Natural history of cervicovaginal papilloma virus infection in young women. N Engl J Med 1998;338:423-8.

Koutsky LA, Kiviat NB. Genital human papillomavirus. In: K. Holmes, P. Sparling, P. Mardh et al (eds). Sexually Transmitted Diseases, 3rd edition. New York: McGraw-Hill, 1999, p. 347-359.

Kiviat NB, Koutsky LA, Paavonen J. Cervical neoplasia and other STD-related genital tract neoplasias. In: K. Holmes, P. Sparling, P. Mardh et al (eds). Sexually Transmitted Diseases, 3rd edition. New York: McGraw-Hill, 1999, p. 811-831.

Myers ER, McCrory DC, Nanda K, Bastian L, Matchar DB. Mathematical model for the natural history of human papillomavirus infection and cervical carcinogenesis. American Journal of Epidemiology 2000; 151(12):1158-1171.

Watts DH, Brunham RC. Sexually transmitted diseases, including HIV infection in pregnancy. In: K. Holmes, P. Sparling, P. Mardh et al (eds). Sexually Transmitted Diseases, 3rd edition. New York: McGraw-Hill, 1999, 1089-1132.

Weinstock H, Berman S, Cates W. Sexually transmitted disease among American youth: Incidence and prevalence estimates, 2000. Perspectives on Sexual and Reproductive Health 2004; 36: 6-10..

Genital Herpes

Results of a nationally representative study show that genital herpes infection is common in the United States. Nationwide, at least 45 million people ages 12 and older, or one out of five adolescents and adults, have had genital HSV infection. Between the late 1970s and the early 1990s, the number of Americans with genital herpes infection increased 30 percent.

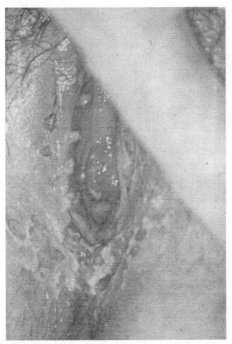

Herpes blisters on the labia and vagina (source CDC STD101 slides)

Genital herpes is caused by the herpes simplex viruses type 1 (HSV-1) and type 2 (HSV-2). Most genital herpes is caused by HSV-2. Most individuals have no or only minimal signs or symptoms from HSV-1 or HSV-2 infection. When signs do occur, they typically appear as one or more blisters on or around the genitals or rectum. The blisters break, leaving tender ulcers (sores) that may take two to four weeks to heal the first time they occur. Typically, another outbreak can appear weeks or months after the first, but it almost always is less severe and shorter than the first outbreak. Although the infection can stay in the body indefinitely, the number of outbreaks tends to decrease over a period of years.

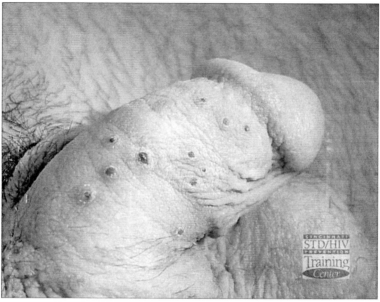
Herpes blisters on the shaft of the penis (source CDC STD101 slides)

Genital HSV-2 infection is more common in women (approximately one out of four women) than in men (almost one out of five). This may be due to male-to-female transmissions being more likely than female-to-male transmission.

HSV-1 and HSV-2 can be found in and released from the sores that the viruses cause, but they also are released between outbreaks from skin that does not appear to be broken or to have a sore. Generally, a person can only get HSV-2 infection during sexual contact with someone who has a genital HSV-2 infection. Transmission can occur from an infected partner who does not have a visible sore and may not know that he or she is infected.

HSV-1 can cause genital herpes, but it more commonly causes infections of the mouth and lips, so-called "fever blisters." HSV-1 infection of the genitals can be caused by oral-genital or genital-

genital contact with a person who has HSV-1 infection. Genital HSV-1 outbreaks recur less regularly than genital HSV-2 outbreaks.

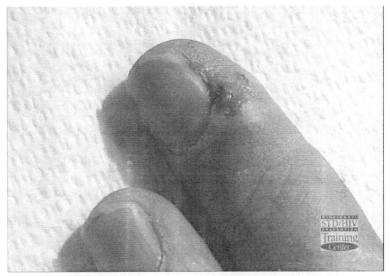

Herpes blister on a finger (source CDC STD101 slides)

Symptoms

Most people infected with HSV-2 are not aware of their infection. However, if signs and symptoms occur during the first outbreak, they can be quite pronounced. The first outbreak usually occurs within two weeks after the virus is transmitted, and the sores typically heal within two to four weeks. Other signs and symptoms during the primary episode may include a second crop of sores, and flu-like symptoms, including fever and swollen glands. However, most individuals with HSV-2 infection may never have sores, or they may have very mild signs that they do not even notice or that they mistake for insect bites or another skin condition.

Most people diagnosed with a first episode of genital herpes can expect to have several (typically four or five) outbreaks (symptomatic recurrences) within a year. Over time these recurrences usually decrease in frequency.

Genital herpes can cause recurrent painful genital sores in many adults, and herpes infection can be severe in people with suppressed immune systems. Regardless of severity of symptoms, genital herpes frequently causes psychological distress in people who know they are infected.

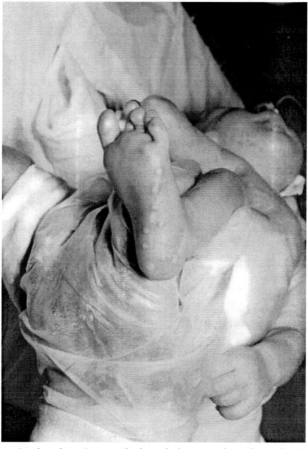

Herpes simplex ulcerations on the lateral plantar surface of an infant's foot.
Women who acquire genital herpes during pregnancy can transmit the virus to their babies. Untreated Herpes Simplex Virus (HSV) infections in newborns can result in mental retardation and death. Source Public Health Image Library (PHIL)

In addition, genital HSV can cause potentially fatal infections in babies. It is important that women avoid contracting herpes during pregnancy because a first episode during pregnancy causes a greater risk of transmission to the baby. If a woman has active genital herpes at delivery, a cesarean delivery is usually performed. Fortunately, infection of a baby from a woman with herpes infection is rare.

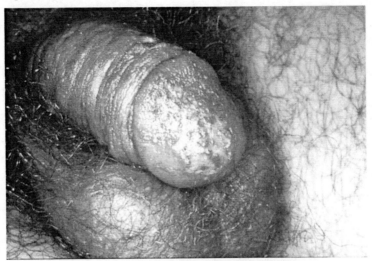

This male presented with primary vesiculopapular herpes genitalis lesions on his glans penis, and penile shaft.

When signs of herpes genitalis do occur, they typically appear as one or more blisters on or around the genitals or rectum. The blisters break, leaving tender ulcers (sores) that may take two to four weeks to heal the first time they occur.
Source PHIL

Herpes may play a role in the spread of HIV, the virus that causes AIDS. Herpes can make people more susceptible to HIV infection, and it can make HIV-infected individuals more infectious.

Diagnosis and Treatment

The signs and symptoms associated with HSV-2 can vary greatly. Health care providers can diagnose genital herpes by visual inspection if the outbreak is typical, and by taking a sample from the sore(s) and testing it in a laboratory. HSV infections can be difficult to diagnose between outbreaks. Blood tests, which detect HSV-1 or HSV-2 infection, may be helpful, although the results are not always clear-cut.

Genital Herpes cannot be "Cured"

There is no treatment that can cure herpes, but antiviral medications can shorten and prevent outbreaks during the period of time the person takes the medication. In addition, daily suppressive therapy for symptomatic herpes can reduce transmission to partners.

The percent of people infected with herpes increases with age because, once infected, people remain infected with this incurable disease throughout their lives. Herpes infection is believed to be acquired most commonly during adolescence and young adulthood, as individuals become sexually active and may have multiple partners.

According to two national surveys between the 1970s and the 1990s, genital herpes increased fastest among white teens ages 12 to 19 years old (Fleming, 1997). Herpes prevalence among white teens ages 12 to 19 years old in the 1990s was five times greater than the prevalence in the 1970s. Among young white adults 20 to 29 years of age, herpes prevalence increased two-fold over that period.

Prevention

The surest way to avoid transmission of sexually transmitted diseases, including genital herpes, is to abstain from sexual contact, or to be in a long-term mutually monogamous relationship with a partner who has been tested and is known to be uninfected.

Genital ulcer diseases can occur in both male and female genital areas that are covered or protected by a latex condom, as well as in areas that are not covered. Correct and consistent use of latex condoms can reduce the risk of genital herpes only when the infected area or site of potential exposure is protected. Since a condom may not cover all infected areas, even correct and consistent use of latex condoms cannot guarantee protection from genital herpes.

Persons with herpes should abstain from sexual activity with uninfected partners when lesions or other symptoms of herpes are present. It is important to know that even if a person does not have any symptoms he or she can still infect sex partners. Sex partners of infected persons should be advised that they may become infected. Sex partners can seek testing to determine if they are infected with HSV. A positive HSV-2 blood test most likely indicates a genital herpes infection.

Sources

Centers for Disease Control and Prevention. Sexually Transmitted Diseases Treatment Guidelines 2002. MMWR 2002;51(no. RR-6)

Centers for Disease Control and Prevention. Sexually Transmitted Disease Surveillance, 2002. Atlanta, GA: U.S. Department of Health and Human Service, October 2003.

Corey L, Wald A. Genital herpes. In: Holmes KK, Sparling PF, Mardh P et al (eds). Sexually Transmitted Disease, 3rd Edition. New York: McGraw-Hill, 1999, p. 285-312.

Corey L, Wald A, Patel R et al. Once-daily valacyclovir to reduce the risk of transmission of genital herpes. New England Journal of Medicine 2004; 350:11-20.

Fleming DT, McQuillan GM, Johnson RE, Nahmias AJ, Aral SO, Lee FK, St. Louis ME. Herpes Simplex Virus Type 2 in the United States, 1976 to 1994. NEJM 1997; 16:1105-1111.

Wald A, Langenberg AGM, Link K, et al. Effect of condoms on reducing the transmission of herpes simplex virus type 2 from men to women. JAMA 2001;285: 3100-3106.

Wald A, Link K. Risk of human immunodeficiency virus infection in herpes simplex virus infection in herpes simplex virus type 2 – seropositive persons: A meta-analysis. J Infect Dis 2002; 185: 45-52.

Weinstock H, Berman S, Cates W. Sexually transmitted diseases among American youth: Incidence and prevalence estimates, 2000. Perspectives on Sexual and Reproductive Health 2004; 36:6-10.

Gonorrhea

Gonorrhea is a very common infectious disease. CDC estimates that more than 700,000 persons in the U.S. get new gonorrheal infections each year. Only about half of these infections are reported to CDC. In 2002, 351,852 cases of gonorrhea were reported to CDC. In the period from 1975 to 1997, the national gonorrhea rate declined, following the implementation of the national gonorrhea control program in the mid-1970s. After a small increase in 1998, the gonorrhea rate has decreased slightly since 1999. In 2002, the rate of reported gonorrheal infections was 125.0 per 100,000 persons.

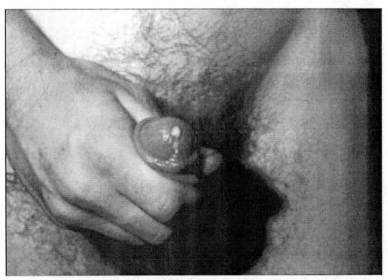

Gonococcal Urethritis with a purulent discharge that may be thick, milky white, yellowish or greenish. Source CDC STD 101

Gonorrhea is caused by Neisseria gonorrhoeae, a bacterium that can grow and multiply easily in the warm, moist areas of the reproductive tract, including the cervix (opening to the womb), uterus (womb), and fallopian tubes (egg canals) in women, and in the urethra (urine canal) in women and men. The bacterium can also grow in the mouth, throat, eyes, and anus.

Gonorrhea is spread through contact with the penis, vagina, mouth, or anus. Ejaculation does not have to occur for gonorrhea to be transmitted or acquired. Gonorrhea can also be spread from mother to baby during delivery.

People who have had gonorrhea and received treatment may get infected again if they have sexual contact with a person infected with gonorrhea.

Any sexually active person can be infected with gonorrhea. In the United States, the highest reported rates of infection are among sexually active teenagers, young adults, and African Americans.

Symptoms

Although many men with gonorrhea may have no symptoms at all, some men have some signs or symptoms that appear two to five days after infection; symptoms can take as long as 30 days to appear. Symptoms and signs include a burning sensation when urinating, or a white, yellow, or green discharge from the penis. Sometimes men with gonorrhea can get epididymitis, a painful condition of the testicles that can lead to infertility if left untreated

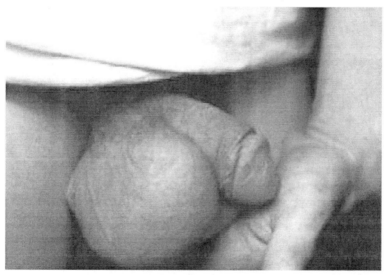

Gonococcal epididymitis with swollen or tender testicles. Source CDC STD101

In women, the symptoms of gonorrhea are often mild, but most women who are infected have no symptoms. Even when a woman has symptoms, they can be so non-specific as to be mistaken for a bladder or vaginal infection. The initial symptoms and signs in women include a painful or burning sensation when urinating, increased vaginal discharge, or vaginal bleeding between periods. Women with gonorrhea are at risk of developing serious complications from the infection, regardless of the presence or severity of symptoms.

Symptoms of rectal infection in both men and women may include discharge, anal itching, soreness, bleeding, or painful bowel movements. Rectal infection also may cause no symptoms. Infections in the throat may cause a sore throat but usually causes no symptoms.

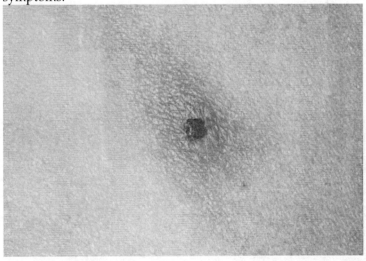

This is a skin lesion in a patient with systemically disseminated *Neisseria gonorrhoeae* bacteria. Gonorrhea, caused by *Neisseria gonorrhoeae*, if left untreated will enter the blood, thereby, spreading throughout the body. As is shown here, such fully systemic dissemination may manifest itself as skin lesions throughout the body. Source PHIL

Untreated gonorrhea can cause serious and permanent health problems in both women and men.

In women, gonorrhea is a common cause of pelvic inflammatory disease (PID). About one million women each year in the

United States develop PID. Women with PID do not necessarily have symptoms. When symptoms are present, they can be very severe and can include abdominal pain and fever. PID can lead to internal abscesses (pus-filled "pockets" that are hard to cure) and long-lasting, chronic pelvic pain. PID can damage the fallopian tubes enough to cause infertility or increase the risk of ectopic pregnancy. Ectopic pregnancy is a life-threatening condition in which a fertilized egg grows outside the uterus, usually in a fallopian tube. See the section on PID.

Gonorrhea can spread to the blood or joints. This condition can be life threatening. In addition, people with gonorrhea can more easily contract HIV, the virus that causes AIDS. HIV-infected people with gonorrhea are more likely to transmit HIV to someone else.

Pregnancy

If a pregnant woman has gonorrhea, she may give the infection to her baby as the baby passes through the birth canal during delivery. This can cause blindness, joint infection, or a life-threatening blood infection in the baby.

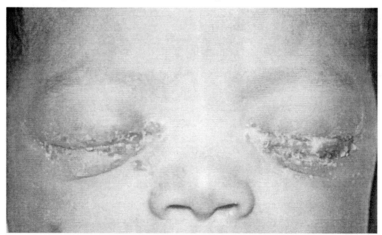

This was a newborn with *gonococcal ophthalmia neonatorum* caused by a maternally transmitted gonococcal infection. Unless preventative measures are taken, it is estimated that *gonococcal ophthalmia neonatorum* will develop in 28% of infants born to women with gonorrhea. It affects the corneal epithelium causing microbial keratitis, ulceration and perforation. Source PHIL

84

Treatment of gonorrhea as soon as it is detected in pregnant women will reduce the risk of these complications. Pregnant women should consult a health care provider for appropriate examination, testing, and treatment, as necessary.

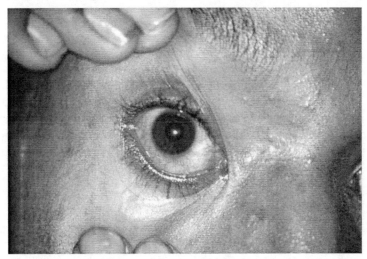

This patient presented with gonococcal urethritis, which became systemically disseminated leading to gonococcal conjunctivitis of the right eye. If untreated *Neisseria gonorrhoeae* bacteria may spread to the bloodstream and, thereby, throughout the body. The most common symptoms are then rash and joint pains, as well such as conjunctivitis, but other generalized symptoms may result. Source PHIL

Diagnosis and Treatment

Several laboratory tests are available to diagnose gonorrhea. A doctor or nurse can obtain a sample for testing from the parts of the body likely to be infected (cervix, urethra, rectum, or throat) and send the sample to a laboratory for analysis. Gonorrhea that is present in the cervix or urethra can be diagnosed in a laboratory by testing a urine sample. A quick laboratory test for gonorrhea that can be done in some clinics or doctor's offices is a Gram stain. A Gram stain of a sample from a urethra or a cervix allows the doctor to see the gonorrhea bacterium under a microscope. This test works better for men than for women.

Several antibiotics can successfully cure gonorrhea in adolescents and adults. However, drug-resistant strains of gonorrhea are increasing in many areas of the world, including the United States, and successful treatment of gonorrhea is becoming more difficult. Because many people with gonorrhea also have chlamydia, another sexually transmitted disease, antibiotics for both infections are usually given together. Persons with gonorrhea should be tested for other STDs.

It is important to take all of the medication prescribed to cure gonorrhea. Although medication will stop the infection, it will not repair any permanent damage done by the disease. People who have had gonorrhea and have been treated can get the disease again if they have sexual contact with persons infected with gonorrhea. If a person's symptoms continue even after receiving treatment, he or she should return to a doctor to be reevaluated.

Prevention

The surest way to avoid transmission of sexually transmitted diseases is to abstain from sexual intercourse, or to be in a long-term mutually monogamous relationship with a partner who has been tested and is known to be uninfected.

Latex condoms, when used consistently and correctly, can reduce the risk of transmission of gonorrhea.

Any genital symptoms such as discharge or burning during urination or unusual sore or rash should be a signal to stop having sex and to see a doctor immediately. If a person has been diagnosed and treated for gonorrhea, he or she should notify all recent sex partners so they can see a health care provider and be treated. This will reduce the risk that the sex partners will develop serious complications from gonorrhea and will also reduce the person's risk of becoming re-infected. The person and all of his or her sex partners must avoid sex until they have completed their treatment for gonorrhea.

Antimicrobial Resistance and Neisseria

Antimicrobial resistance in N. gonorrhoeae remains an important challenge to controlling gonorrhea; gonococcal strains may be resistant to penicillins, tetracyclines, spectinomycin, and fluoroquinolones. Resistance to CDC-recommended doses of ciprofloxacin and ofloxacin exceeds 40% in some Asian countries (World Health Organization (WHO) Western Pacific Region Gonococcal Antimicrobial Susceptibility Programme (GASP) Report- 2000. Commun Dis Intell 2001; 25:274-277).

Fluoroquinolone-resistant strains of N. gonorrhoeae have also been reported in the United States and Canada. The proportion of gonococcal isolates in Hawaii that are fluoroquinolone-resistant currently exceeds 13% and increasing numbers of resistant strains have been identified in the continental United States (Gonococcal Isolate Surveillance Project (GISP) Annual Report - 2003).

Antimicrobial resistance in N. gonorrhoeae occurs as plasmid-mediated resistance to penicillin and tetracycline, and chromosomally mediated resistance to penicillins, tetracyclines, spectinomycin, and fluoroquinolones.

Surveillance

Surveillance for antimicrobial resistance in N. gonorrhoeae in the United States is conducted through the Gonococcal Isolate Surveillance Project (GISP). The Gonococcal Isolate Surveillance Project (GISP) was established in 1986 to monitor trends in antimicrobial susceptibilities of strains of N. gonorrhoeae in the United States and to establish a rational basis for the selection of gonococcal therapies. Approximately 26 cities participate in GISP. Data from this project have been reported and used to revise the CDC's STD Treatment Guidelines in 1989, 1993, 1998, and 2002.

Trends

Antimicrobial resistance remains an important consideration in the treatment of gonorrhea. Overall, 16.4%of isolates collected in 2003 by GISP were resistant to penicillin, tetracycline, or both. The percentage of GISP isolates that were penicillinase-producing Neisseria gonorrhoeae (PPNG) declined from a peak of 11.0% in 1991 to 1.0% in 2003. In contrast, the percentage of isolates with chromosomally mediated resistance to penicillin (PenR) had increased from 0.5% in 1988 to 5.7% in 1999 and then declined to 1.3% in 2003. The prevalence of chromosomally mediated tetracycline resistance (TetR) decreased every year since 1995, until 2002, when it slightly increased. In 2003 there was another slight increase to 6.2%. The prevalence of isolates with chromosomally mediated resistance to penicillin and tetracycline (CMRNG) increased from 3.0% in 1989 to a peak of 8.7% in 1997 and declined to 3.8% in 2003.

Resistance to ciprofloxacin was first identified in GISP in 1991. From 1991 to 1998, fewer than 9 ciprofloxacin-resistant isolates were identified each year and such isolates were identified in only a few GISP clinics. In 2000, similar to 1999, 19 (0.4%) ciprofloxacin-resistant GISP isolates were identified in 7 of the 25 GISP clinics. In 2001, 38 (0.7%) ciprofloxacin-resistant GISP isolates were identified in 6 clinics. Two hundred seventy (4.1%) of GISP isolates were resistant to ciprofloxacin (MICs >1.0 g/ml) in 2003, which was two times the proportion identified in 2002 (2.2%, 116/5367). Ciprofloxacin-resistant isolates were identified in 70% (21/30) sentinel sites in 2003.

In 2003, no GISP isolates had decreased susceptibility to cefixime or ceftriaxone. The proportion of GISP isolates demonstrating decreased susceptibility to ceftriaxone or cefixime has remained very low over time. To date, no cephalosporin resistance has been identified in GISP. However, it was notable that three of the four isolates with decreased susceptibility to cefixime were also resistant to penicillin, tetracycline, and ciprofloxacin; such multi-drug resistance in combination with decreased susceptibility to cefixime has rarely been identified in the United States (Wang SA, Lee MV, Iverson CJ, O'Connor N, Ohye RG, Hale JA, Knapp JS, Effler PV, Weinstock HS. Multi-drug resistant Neisseria gonorrhoeae with decreased susceptibility to cefixime, Hawaii 2001. [Abstract] International Conference on Emerging Infectious Diseases, Atlanta, Georgia, March 25, 2002.) [Note: no NCCLS criteria currently exist for resistance of N. gonorrhoeae to cephalosporins].

The proportion of GISP isolates demonstrating elevated minimum inhibitory concentrations (MICs) to azithromycin has been increasing since GISP began monitoring azithromycin susceptibility in 1992. In 1992, 0.9% of GISP isolates had azithromycin MIC 0.5 µg/ml compared with 2.2% in 2003. In 1992, there were no isolates with azithromycin MIC 1.0 µg/ml, but in 2003 there were 26 such isolates. [Note: no NCCLS criteria currently exist for susceptibility or resistance of N. gonorrhoeae to azithromycin].

Challenges and Ongoing work

Major challenges to monitoring antimicrobial resistance of N. gonorrhoeae include substantial declines in the use of gonorrhea culture for testing and declines in the number of laboratories performing gonorrhea susceptibility testing. There has been a proliferation of non-culture diagnostic testing for gonorrhea. In many clinical settings, non-culture testing has completely replaced testing using culture. Currently, susceptibility testing can only be performed on N. gonorrhoeae growing in culture. Technology that allows susceptibility testing from non-culture specimens is needed. Research into determining mechanisms of resistance for the newer antimicrobials and for determining the upper limits of resistance conferred by currently recognized mechanisms of resistance to fluoroquinolones is ongoing.

Research into determining mechanisms of resistance for the newer antimicrobials and for determining the upper limits of resistance conferred by currently recognized mechanisms of resistance to fluoroquinolones is ongoing.

CDC conducts national surveillance for antimicrobial resistance in N. gonorrhoeae via GISP and performs outbreak investigations of resistant gonococcal infections as needed. CDC also performs laboratory confirmation for clinicians who identify or suspect antimicrobial resistance in patients with gonorrhea. CDC publishes updated STD Treatment Guidelines on a regular basis to guide use of appropriate and effective antimicrobial therapy for gonorrhea and other STD treatment.

Sources

Centers for Disease Control and Prevention. Sexually Transmitted Diseases Treatment Guidelines 2002. MMWR 2002;51(no. RR-6)

Centers for Disease Control and Prevention. Sexually Transmitted Disease Surveillance, 2002. Atlanta, GA: U.S. Department of Health and Human Service, October 2003.

Hook, E.W. III and Handsfield, H.H. Gonococcal infections in the adult. In: K. Holmes, P. Markh, P. Sparling et al (eds). Sexually Transmitted Diseases, 3rd Edition. New York: McGraw-Hill, 1999, 451-466.

Weinstock H, Berman S, Cates W. Sexually transmitted disease among American youth: Incidence and prevalence estimates, 2000. Perspectives on Sexual and Reproductive Health 2004; 36: 6-10.

Pelvic inflammatory disease

Each year in the United States, it is estimated that more than 1 million women experience an episode of acute PID. More than 100,000 women become infertile each year as a result of PID, and a large proportion of the ectopic pregnancies occurring every year are due to the consequences of PID. Annually more than 150 women die from PID or its complications.

Pelvic inflammatory disease (PID) is a general term that refers to infection of the uterus (womb), fallopian tubes (tubes that carry eggs from the ovaries to the uterus) and other reproductive organs. It is a common and serious complication of some sexually transmitted diseases (STDs), especially chlamydia and gonorrhea. PID can damage the fallopian tubes and tissues in and near the uterus and ovaries. Untreated PID can lead to serious consequences including infertility, ectopic pregnancy (a pregnancy in the fallopian tube or elsewhere outside of the womb), abscess formation, and chronic pelvic pain.

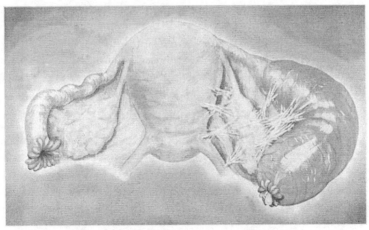

Pelvic Inflammatory Disease. Source CDC STD101

PID occurs when bacteria move upward from a woman's vagina or cervix (opening to the uterus) into her reproductive organs. Many different organisms can cause PID, but many cases are associated with gonorrhea and chlamydia, two very common bacterial STDs. A prior episode of PID increases the risk of another episode because the reproductive organs may be damaged during the initial bout of infection.

Sexually active women in their childbearing years are most at risk, and those under age 25 are more likely to develop PID than those older than 25. This is because the cervix of teenage girls and young women is not fully matured, increasing their susceptibility to the STDs that are linked to PID.

The more sex partners a woman has, the greater her risk of developing PID. Also, a woman whose partner has more than one sex partner is at greater risk of developing PID, because of the potential for more exposure to infectious agents.

Women who douche may have a higher risk of developing PID compared with women who do not douche. Research has shown that douching changes the vaginal flora (organisms that live in the vagina) in harmful ways, and can force bacteria into the upper reproductive organs from the vagina.

Women who have an intrauterine device (IUD) inserted may have a slightly increased risk of PID near the time of insertion compared with women using other contraceptives or no contraceptive at all. However, this risk is greatly reduced if a woman is tested and, if necessary, treated for STDs before an IUD is inserted.

Symptoms

Symptoms of PID vary from none to severe. When PID is caused by chlamydial infection, a woman may experience mild symptoms or no symptoms at all, while serious damage is being done to her reproductive organs. Because of vague symptoms, PID goes unrecognized by women and their health care providers about two thirds of the time. Women who have symptoms of PID most commonly have lower abdominal pain. Other signs and symptoms include fever, unusual vaginal discharge that may have a foul odor, painful intercourse, painful urination, irregular menstrual bleeding, and pain in the right upper abdomen (rare).

Prompt and appropriate treatment can help prevent complications of PID. Without treatment, PID can cause permanent damage to the female reproductive organs. Infection-causing bacteria can silently invade the fallopian tubes, causing normal tissue to turn into scar tissue. This scar tissue blocks or interrupts the normal movement of eggs into the uterus. If the fallopian tubes are totally blocked by scar tissue, sperm cannot fertilize an egg, and the woman becomes infertile. Infertility also can occur if the fallopian tubes are partially blocked or even slightly damaged. About one in eight women with PID becomes infertile, and if a woman has multiple episodes of PID, her chances of becoming infertile increase.

In addition, a partially blocked or slightly damaged fallopian tube may cause a fertilized egg to remain in the fallopian tube. If this fertilized egg begins to grow in the tube as if it were in the uterus, it is called an ectopic pregnancy. As it grows, an ectopic pregnancy can rupture the fallopian tube causing severe pain, internal bleeding, and even death.

Scarring in the fallopian tubes and other pelvic structures can also cause chronic pelvic pain (pain that lasts for months or even years). Women with repeated episodes of PID are more likely to suffer infertility, ectopic pregnancy, or chronic pelvic pain.

Diagnosis and Treatment

PID is difficult to diagnose because the symptoms are often subtle and mild. Many episodes of PID go undetected because the woman or her health care provider fails to recognize the implications of mild or nonspecific symptoms. Because there are no precise tests for PID, a diagnosis is usually based on clinical findings. If symptoms such as lower abdominal pain are present, a health care provider should perform a physical examination to determine the nature and location of the pain and check for fever, abnormal vaginal or cervical discharge, and for evidence of gonorrheal or chlamydial infection. If the findings suggest PID, treatment is necessary.

The health care provider may also order tests to identify the infection-causing organism (e.g., chlamydial or gonorrheal infection) or to distinguish between PID and other problems with similar symptoms. A pelvic ultrasound is a helpful procedure for diagnosing PID. An ultrasound can view the pelvic area to see whether the fallopian tubes are enlarged or whether an abscess is present. In some cases, a laparoscopy may be necessary to confirm the diagnosis. A laparoscopy is a minor surgical procedure in which a thin, flexible tube with a lighted end (laparoscope) is inserted through a small incision in the lower abdomen. This procedure enables the doctor to view the internal pelvic organs and to take specimens for laboratory studies, if needed.

PID can be cured with several types of antibiotics. A health care provider will determine and prescribe the best therapy. However, antibiotic treatment does not reverse any damage that has already occurred to the reproductive organs. If a woman has pelvic pain and other symptoms of PID, it is critical that she seek care immediately. Prompt antibiotic treatment can prevent severe damage to reproductive organs. The longer a woman delays treatment for PID, the more likely she is to become infertile or to have a future ectopic pregnancy because of damage to the fallopian tubes.

Because of the difficulty in identifying organisms infecting the internal reproductive organs and because more than one organism may be responsible for an episode of PID, PID is usually treated with at least two antibiotics that are effective against a wide range of infectious agents. These antibiotics can be given by mouth or by injection. The symptoms may go away before the infection is cured. Even if symptoms go away, the woman should finish taking all of the prescribed medicine. This will help prevent the infection from returning. Women being treated for PID should be re-evaluated by their health care provider two to three days after starting treatment to be sure the antibiotics are working to cure the infection. In addition, a woman's sex partner(s) should be treated to decrease the risk of re-infection, even if the partner(s) has no symptoms. Although sex partners may have no symptoms, they may still be infected with the organisms that can cause PID.

Hospitalization to treat PID may be recommended if the woman (1) is severely ill (e.g., nausea, vomiting, and high fever); (2) is pregnant; (3) does not respond to or cannot take oral medication and needs intravenous antibiotics; or (4) has an abscess in the fallopian tube or ovary (tubo-ovarian abscess). If symptoms continue or if an abscess does not go away, surgery may be needed. Complications of PID, such as chronic pelvic pain and scarring are difficult to treat, but sometimes they improve with surgery.

Prevention

STD (mainly untreated Chlamydia or gonorrhea) is the main preventable cause of PID. Women can protect themselves from PID by taking action to prevent STDs or by getting early treatment if they do get an STD.

The surest way to avoid transmission of STDs is to abstain from sexual intercourse, or to be in a long-term mutually monogamous relationship with a partner who has been tested and is known to be uninfected.

Latex male condoms, when used consistently and correctly, can reduce the risk of transmission of chlamydia and gonorrhea.

CDC recommends yearly chlamydia testing of all sexually active women age 25 or younger and of older women with risk factors for chlamydial infections (those who have a new sex partner or multiple sex partners). An appropriate sexual risk assessment by a health care provider should always be conducted and may indicate more frequent screening for some women.

Any genital symptoms such as an unusual sore, discharge with odor, burning during urination, or bleeding between menstrual cycles could mean an STD infection. If a woman has any of these symptoms, she should stop having sex and consult a health care provider immediately. Treating STDs early can prevent PID. Women who are told they have an STD and are treated for it should notify all of their recent sex partners so they can see a health care provider and be evaluated for STDs. Sexual activity should not resume until all sex partners have been examined and, if necessary, treated.

Sources

American College of Obstetricians and Gynecologists (ACOG). Pelvic Inflammatory Disease. ACOG Patient Education Pamphlet, 1999.

Centers for Disease Control and Prevention. Sexually transmitted diseases treatment guidelines 2002. MMWR 2002;51(no. RR-6).

Westrom, L and Eschenbach, D. Chapter 58 In: K. Holmes, P. Mardh, P. Sparling et al (eds). Sexually Transmitted Diseases, 3rd Edition. New York: McGraw-Hill, 1999, 783-809.

Hepatitis

Hepatitis is an inflammation of the liver caused by certain viruses and other factors, such as alcohol abuse, some medications, and trauma. Its various forms affect millions of Americans. Although many cases of hepatitis are not a serious threat to health, the disease can become chronic (long-lasting) and can sometimes lead to liver failure and death.

Cause

There are four major types of viral hepatitis:

Hepatitis A, caused by infection with the hepatitis A virus, is usually a mild disease that does not become chronic. The virus is sometimes passed on through sexual practices involving oral-anal contact. It is most commonly spread by food and water contamination

Hepatitis B, caused by infection with the hepatitis B virus (HBV), may be mild or severe, acute or chronic. HBV is most commonly passed on to a sexual partner during intercourse, especially during anal sex. Because the disease is not easily spread, persons with HBV should not worry about spreading it through casual contact such as shaking hands or sharing a workspace or bathroom facility.

Each year, an estimated 300,000 persons in the United States become infected with HBV. Hepatitis B is most commonly transmitted by sharing drug needles, by engaging in high-risk sexual behavior, from a mother to her newborn, and in the health care setting.

Non-A, non-B hepatitis is primarily caused by the hepatitis C virus (HCV). Although generally a mild condition, it is much more likely than hepatitis B to lead to chronic liver disease. HCV appears to be spread through sexual contact as well as through sharing drug needles. Sexual spread, however, is inefficient and much less than that for HBV or the AIDS virus (HIV). With the advent of new tests to screen blood donors, a very small percentage of persons with HCV currently become infected through blood transfusions. The hepatitis E virus causes another type of non-A, non-B hepatitis. This virus is principally spread through contaminated water in areas with poor sanitation. This form of hepatitis does not occur in the U.S. and is not known to be passed on through sexual contact.

Delta hepatitis occurs only in people who already are infected with HBV. A potentially severe disease, it is caused by a virus (HDV) that can produce disease only when HBV is also present. Most cases occur among people who are frequently exposed to blood and blood products, such as people with hemophilia. Small-scale epidemics have occurred among injection drug users who share contaminated needles.

Experts believe that HDV may be sexually transmitted, but further research is needed to provide more specific evidence.

Transmission

HBV, HCV, and HDV can be spread in the following ways:

- Having sexual intercourse with an infected person without using a condom.
- Sharing drug needles among users of injected street drugs.
- Needle-stick accidents among health-care workers.
- Mother-to-child transmission of HBV during birth.
- Transfusions. Until recently, blood transfusions were the most frequent cause of hepatitis C. Blood banks in the United States now screen donated blood for HBV and HCV and discard any blood that appears to be infected. Therefore, the risk of acquiring hepatitis from these viruses is very low in the U.S. and in other countries where blood is similarly tested. Tests to screen blood for HBV will also screen out HDV.
- Personal contact with an infected person. HBV, HCV, and HDV sometimes spread when household

members unknowingly come in contact with virus-infected blood or body fluids--most probably through cuts and scrapes or by sharing personal items such as razors and toothbrushes. While it is possible to become infected by contact with saliva, blood and semen remain the major sources of infection.

Symptoms

Many people infected with viral hepatitis have no symptoms. For example, about one-third of people infected with HBV have a completely "silent" disease. When symptoms are present, they may be mild or severe. The most common early symptoms are mild fever, headache, muscle aches, fatigue, loss of appetite, nausea, vomiting, or diarrhea. Later symptoms may include dark and foamy urine and pale feces; abdominal pain; and yellowing of the skin and whites of the eyes (jaundice).

About 15 to 20 percent of patients develop short-term arthritis-like problems as part of a more severe case of hepatitis B. Another one-third of those with hepatitis B develop only mild flu-like symptoms without jaundice. Very severe (fulminant) hepatitis B is rare, but life-threatening. Early signs of fulminant hepatitis, such as personality changes and agitated behavior, require immediate medical attention.

Some people infected with HBV or HCV become chronic carriers of the virus, although they may have no symptoms. There are an estimated 1.5 million HBV carriers in the U.S. and 300 million carriers worldwide. Children are at greatest risk. About 90 percent of babies who become infected at birth with HBV, and up to half of youngsters who are infected before age 5, become chronic carriers. It is estimated that there are between 2 and 5 million HCV chronic carriers. At least half of all HCV carriers will develop chronic liver disease, regardless of whether or not they have symptoms.

Diagnosis

Hepatitis B. Several types of blood tests can detect signs of HBV even before symptoms develop. These tests measure liver function and identify HBV antigens (proteins of the virus) or antibodies (proteins produced by the body in response to the virus) in the blood.

Tests for hepatitis B include:

Hepatitis B Surface Antigen (HBsAg). Most people with acute hepatitis B have HBsAg in their blood before symptoms develop. As a person recovers from the illness, HBsAg disappears. If it is still present 6 months after infection, it may indicate that a person has developed chronic hepatitis or may be a symptomless carrier of the virus. HBsAg can be detected by a number of laboratory tests such as radioimmunoassay or enzyme-linked immunosorbent assay (ELISA). Antibody to the surface antigen (anti-HBs) persists for many years. This antibody usually appears as the acute illness improves, providing protection against future HBV infections.

Diagram of Hepatitis B Virus

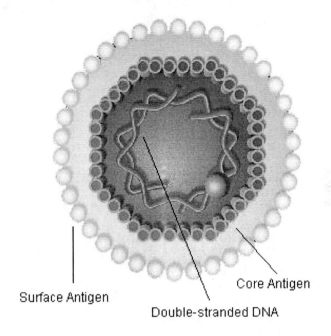

Surface Antigen

Double-stranded DNA

Core Antigen

Hepatitis B Core Antigen (HBcAg). The HBV core protein can be identified only after the surface antigen has been stripped away using special techniques. Commercially available blood tests cannot detect HBcAg in blood, but antibody to the core antigen (anti-HBc) can be detected during acute illness. High levels of anti-HBc are present at the start of illness, and they gradually decrease over time in most people. In contrast, chronic carriers of HBV have high levels of anti-HBc in their blood that may persist throughout life.

E Antigen (HBeAg). The presence of e antigen indicates that a person infected with HBV is highly infectious. An HBsAg-positive pregnant woman whose blood contains e antigen is likely to transmit the virus to her newborn. By contrast, antibody to the e antigen (anti-HBe) may point to a lower degree of infectivity and a reduced likelihood of becoming a carrier. Laboratory blood tests can detect e antigen as well as anti-HBe.

Liver Function Tests. A number of blood tests can be performed to determine how well a person's liver is functioning, and these results can aid in diagnosing hepatitis B infection. High levels of the liver enzymes aspartate transferase (AST) and alanine transferase (ALT) are of particular importance. (These were formerly called SGOT and SGPT.)

Delta hepatitis. Until recently, delta hepatitis could be diagnosed only by liver biopsy in which a tiny piece of the liver is removed and examined. Scientists have developed a procedure to detect part of the genetic material of the virus in a patient's blood, which will allow easier, faster diagnosis. A blood test is also now available to detect antibody to delta antigen (a protein found inside the delta hepatitis virus).

Hepatitis C. A new test is now available to detect hepatitis C. The test identifies antibody to HCV, which is present in more than 50 percent of persons with acute hepatitis C and in almost all with chronic hepatitis.

Treatment

At present, there are no specific treatments for the acute symptoms of viral hepatitis. Doctors recommend bed rest, a healthy diet, and avoidance of alcoholic beverages to reduce stress on the liver.

A genetically engineered form of a naturally occurring protein, interferon alpha, is used to treat people with chronic hepatitis C. Studies supported by the National Institutes of Health (NIH) led to the approval of interferon alpha for the treatment of those with chronic HBV as well. The drug improves liver function in some people with hepatitis and diminishes symptoms, although it may cause side effects such as headache, fever, and other flu-like symptoms. Some patients do not respond to interferon alpha, and in others its beneficial effects lessen over time. Scientists are evaluating a number of experimental therapies that may be more effective and less toxic.

Possible Complications

Most patients with mild to severe acute hepatitis begin to feel better in 2 to 3 weeks and recover completely within 4 to 8 weeks. People with acute HBV infection who develop an HCV infection at the same time may be at particular risk for developing severe, life-threatening acute hepatitis.

Many chronic carriers remain symptom free or develop only a mild condition, chronic persistent hepatitis. However, a small percentage go on to develop the most serious complications of viral hepatitis: cirrhosis of the liver, liver cancer, and immune system disorders. Chronic carriers of HBV who become infected with HDV may develop severe acute hepatitis. They also have a high risk of becoming carriers of HDV.

Prevention

The most effective means of preventing viral hepatitis is to avoid contact with the blood, saliva, semen, or vaginal secretions of infected individuals. People who have acute or chronic viral hepatitis should:

Avoid sharing items that could infect others, such as razors or toothbrushes.

Protect sex partners from exposure to their semen, vaginal fluids, or blood. Properly used condoms may be effective in preventing sexual transmission.

There are several vaccines available to prevent hepatitis B. People at high risk of infection should consider vaccination: male homosexuals and heterosexuals with multiple partners, people who receive hemodialysis or blood products, household and sexual contacts of HBV carriers, and users of intravenous street drugs who share needles. Regulations now require health care and laboratory workers who handle blood and other body fluids to be vaccinated. People who have come into direct contact with the blood or body fluids of an HBV carrier may receive one or more injections of hepatitis B immune globulin, sometimes in combination with hepatitis B vaccine. Immune globulin offers temporary protection, while the vaccine provides a longer-lasting immunity.

In an effort to eliminate chronic carriers, the U.S. Centers for Disease Control recommends that all newborn babies be vaccinated. Other groups have recommended that pregnant women be screened for HBsAg as part of their routine prenatal care. If they are infected, their babies can be given hepatitis B immune globulin as well as vaccine immediately after birth.

No vaccines yet exist for HCV or HDV; however, HBV vaccine will prevent delta hepatitis as well.

Research

NIAID supported scientists are attacking hepatitis infection from several fronts. Work is under way to evaluate the potential of antiviral drugs to treat people already infected with HBV, HCV, and HDV. Vaccines and drugs are being tested in the woodchuck, an animal that develops a disease similar to HBV infection in humans. This animal also can be a chronic carrier of HDV, making it a valuable model for studying these viruses and helping scientists understand hepatitis infection.

In addition to testing their effectiveness, scientists are studying how to make antiviral drugs less toxic and how to deliver them to their appropriate targets in the body.

By studying the immune response to hepatitis viruses, scientists hope to identify the precise mechanisms that lead to either recovery or chronic disease. Knowledge is being gained from studies with transgenic mice (mice that carry human genes for HBV). By modifying viral genes and inoculating pregnant women, it may be possible to boost the immune response of babies to HBV. This approach could reduce a large number of chronic carriers and stem the spread of the disease to future generations.

Syphilis

In the United States, health officials reported over 32,000 cases of syphilis in 2002, including 6,862 cases of primary and secondary (P&S) syphilis. In 2002, half of all P&S syphilis cases were reported from 16 counties and 1 city; and most P&S syphilis cases occurred in persons 20 to 39 years of age. The incidence of infectious syphilis was highest in women 20 to 24 years of age and in men 35 to 39 years of age. Reported cases of congenital syphilis in newborns decreased from 2001 to 2002, with 492 new cases reported in 2001 compared to 412 cases in 2002.

Between 2001 and 2002, the number of reported P & S syphilis cases increased 12.4 percent. Rates in women continued to decrease, and overall, the rate in men was 3.5 times that in women. This, in conjunction with reports of syphilis outbreaks in men who have sex with men (MSM), suggests that rates of syphilis in MSM are increasing. Over the past several years, increases in syphilis among MSM have been reported in various cities and areas, including Chicago, Seattle, San Francisco, Southern California, Miami, and New York City. In the recent outbreaks, high rates of HIV co-infection were documented, ranging from 20 percent to 70 percent. While the health problems caused by syphilis in adults are serious in their own right, it is now known that the genital sores caused by syphilis in adults also make it easier to transmit and acquire HIV infection sexually.

Syphilis is caused by the bacterium Treponema pallidum. It has often been called "the great imitator" because so many of the signs and symptoms are indistinguishable from those of other diseases.

Syphilis is passed from person to person through direct contact with a syphilis sore. Sores occur mainly on the external genitals, vagina, anus, or in the rectum. Sores also can occur on the lips and in the mouth. Transmission of the organism occurs during vaginal, anal, or oral sex. Pregnant women with the disease can pass it to the babies they are carrying. Syphilis cannot be spread through contact with toilet seats, doorknobs, swimming pools, hot tubs, bathtubs, shared clothing, or eating utensils.

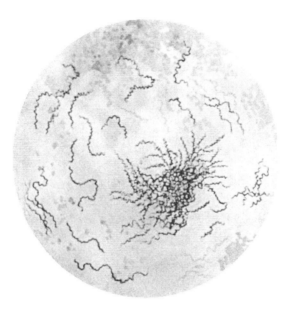

A photomicrograph of *Treponema pallidum* bacteria using Fontana stain. Syphilis is passed from person to person through direct contact with a syphilis sore containing *T. pallidum* bacteria, and occurring mainly on the external genitals, vagina, anus, or in the rectum. Source PHIL

Symptoms

Many people infected with syphilis do not have any symptoms for years, yet remain at risk for late complications if they are not treated. Although transmission appears to occur from persons with sores who are in the primary or secondary stage, many of these sores are unrecognized. Thus, most transmission is from persons who are unaware of their infection.

Primary Stage

The primary stage of syphilis is usually marked by the appearance of a single sore (called a chancre), but there may be multiple sores. The time between infection with syphilis and the start of the first symptom can range from 10 to 90 days (average 21 days). The chancre is usually firm, round, small, and painless. It appears at the spot where syphilis entered the body. The chancre lasts 3 to 6 weeks, and it heals without treatment. However, if adequate treatment is not administered, the infection progresses to the secondary stage.

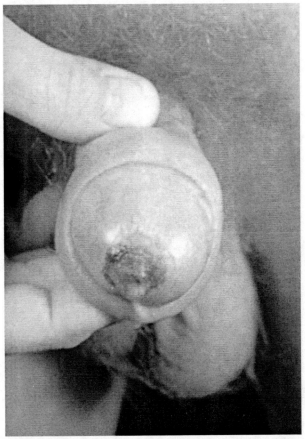

Photograph of a primary syphilitic penile meatal chancre caused by the bacterium *Treponema pallidum*. This patient has a primary syphilitic chancre located in the urethral meatus. A chancre is a primary skin lesion of syphilis which begins at the site of infection after an interval of 10-30 days as a papule or red ulcerated skin lesion. Source PHIL

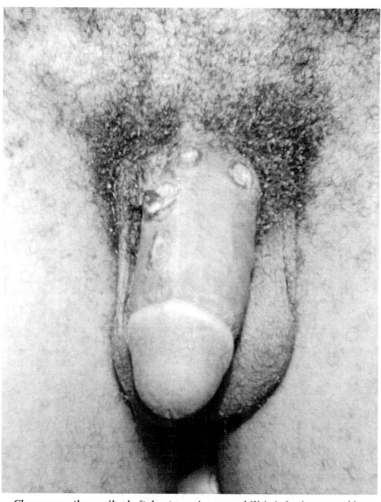

Chancres on the penile shaft due to a primary syphilitic infection caused by *Treponema pallidum* **bacteria.** The primary stage of syphilis is usually marked by the appearance of a single sore called a chancre. The chancre is usually firm, round, small, and painless. Source PHIL

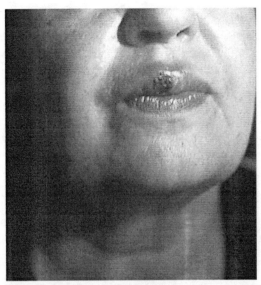

-This patient presented with an extragenital facial chancre of the lip. The primary stage of syphilis is usually marked by the appearance of a sore called a chancre. The chancre is usually firm, round, small, and painless. It appears at the spot where syphilis entered the body, and lasts 3-6 weeks, healing on its own. Source PHIL

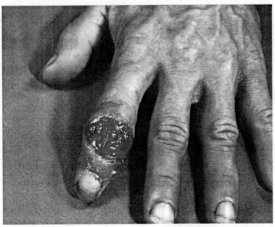

This patient presented with an extragenital syphilitic chancre of the left index finger. The chancre is usually firm, round, small, and painless, appearing at the spot where syphilis entered the body, and lasts 3-6 weeks, healing on its own. If adequate treatment is not administered, the infection progresses to the secondary stage. Source PHIL

Secondary Stage

Skin rash and mucous membrane lesions characterize the secondary stage. This stage typically starts with the development of a rash on one or more areas of the body. The rash usually does not cause itching. Rashes associated with secondary syphilis can appear as the chancre is healing or several weeks after the chancre has healed. The characteristic rash of secondary syphilis may appear as rough, red, or reddish brown spots both on the palms of the hands and the bottoms of the feet. However, rashes with a different appearance may occur on other parts of the body, sometimes resembling rashes caused by other diseases. Sometimes rashes associated with secondary syphilis are so faint that they are not noticed.

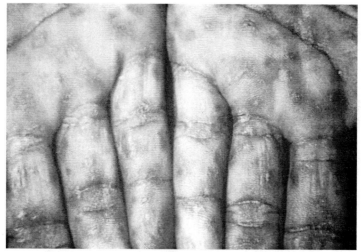

This photograph shows a close-up view of keratotic lesions on the palms of this patient's hands due to a secondary syphilitic infection. Syphilis is a complex sexually transmitted disease (STD) caused by the bacterium *Treponema pallidum*. It has often been called "the great imitator" because so many of the signs and symptoms are indistinguishable from those of other diseases. Source PHIL

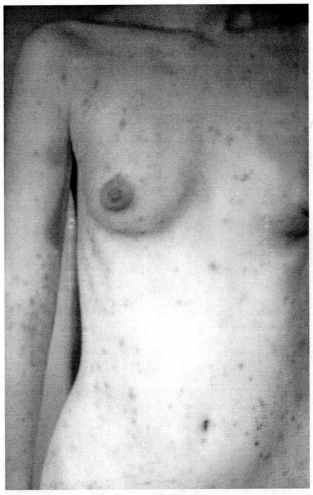

A photograph of a secondary syphilitic papulosquamous rash seen on the torso and upper body. This patient had an extensive papulosquamous rash that developed during secondary syphilis. The rash often appears as rough, red or reddish brown spots that can appear on palms of hands, soles of feet, the chest and back, or other parts of the body. Source PHIL

In addition to rashes, symptoms of secondary syphilis may include fever, swollen lymph glands, sore throat, patchy hair loss, headaches, weight loss, muscle aches, and fatigue. The signs and symptoms of secondary syphilis will resolve with or without treatment, but without treatment, the infection will progress to the latent and late stages of disease.

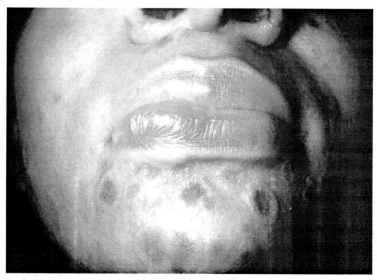

A photograph of a patient with secondary syphilis showing typical "nickel and dime" lesions on the face. A patient with typical "nickel and dime" lesions on the face, which can develop during secondary syphilis. Other symptoms that may occur during this stage are mild fever, fatigue, headache, sore throat, patchy hair loss, and swollen lymph glands. Source PHIL

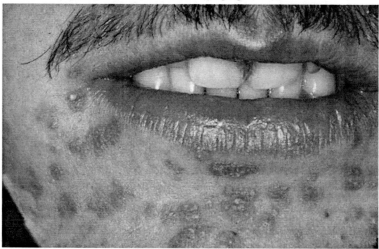

Secondary Syphilis rash on the face. Source CDC STD101

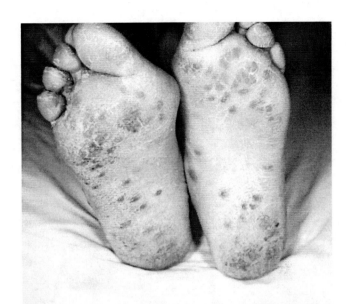

This patient presented with a papulosquamous rash of secondary syphilitic lesions on the plantar surface of his feet. The second stage starts when one or more areas of the skin break into a rash that appears as rough, red or reddish brown spots both on the palms of the hands and on the bottoms of the feet. Even without treatment, rashes clear up on their own. Source PHIL

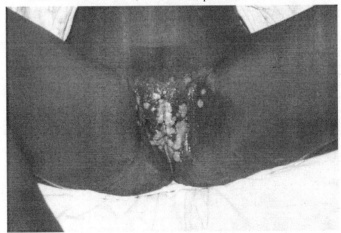

This patient presented with condylomata lata lesions involving the vulva and anal region. A patient with condylomata lata can develop lesions during secondary syphilis, which present as gray, raised papules appearing on the vulva and near the anus, or in any other warm intertriginous region. Source PHIL

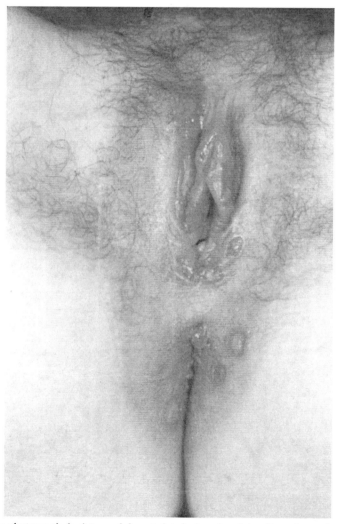

This photograph depicts condylomata lata lesions involving the vulva and anal region. This patient presented with condylomata lata lesions, which present as gray, raised papules appearing on the vulva and near the anus, or in any other warm intertriginous region. Source PHIL

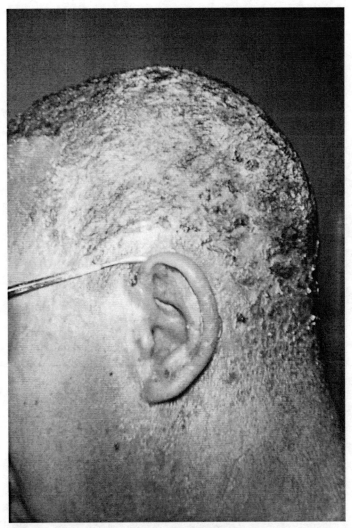

This patient presented with what was first thought to be syphilis, but turned out to be seborrheic dermatitis. Syphilis is a complex sexually transmitted disease (STD) caused by the bacterium *Treponema pallidum*. It has often been called "the great imitator" because so many of the signs and symptoms are indistinguishable from those of other diseases. Source PHIL

Late Stage

The latent (hidden) stage of syphilis begins when secondary symptoms disappear. Without treatment, the infected person will continue to have syphilis even though there are no signs or symptoms; infection remains in the body.

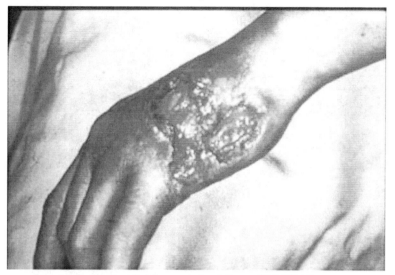

Tertiary Syphilis Ulcer on the hand. Source CDC STD101

In the late stages of syphilis, it may subsequently damage the internal organs, including the brain, nerves, eyes, heart, blood vessels, liver, bones, and joints. This internal damage may show up many years later. Signs and symptoms of the late stage of syphilis include difficulty coordinating muscle movements, paralysis, numbness, gradual blindness, and dementia. This damage may be serious enough to cause death.

Syphilis and Pregnancy

The syphilis bacterium can infect the baby of a woman during her pregnancy. Depending on how long a pregnant woman has been infected, she may have a high risk of having a stillbirth (a baby born dead) or of giving birth to a baby who dies shortly after birth. An infected baby may be born without signs or symptoms of disease. However, if not treated immediately, the baby may develop serious problems within a few weeks. Untreated babies may become developmentally delayed, have seizures, or die.

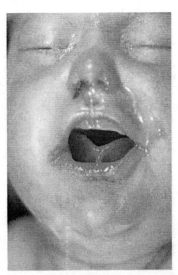

The face of a newborn infant displaying pathologic morphology indicative of "Congenital Syphilis". A pregnant woman with syphilis can pass *T. pallidum* to her unborn child, who may be born with serious mental and physical problems as a result of this infection. When a newborn is affected it is known as "Congenital Syphilis". Source PHIL

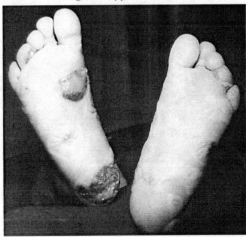

This was a case of congenital syphilis resulting in the death of this newborn infant. Depending on how long a pregnant woman has been infected, she has a good chance of having a stillbirth, known as "syphilitic stillbirth", or of giving birth to a baby who dies shortly after birth. Source PHIL

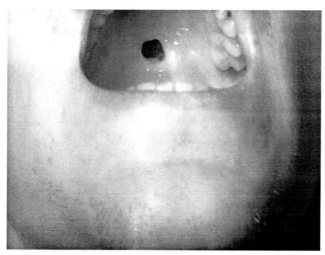

This photograph depicts a perforated hard palate on a patient with congenital syphilis. This patient with congenital syphilis has developed a perforation of hard palate due to gummatous destruction. These destructive tumors can also attack the skin, long bones, eyes, mucous membranes, throat, liver, or stomach lining. Source PHIL

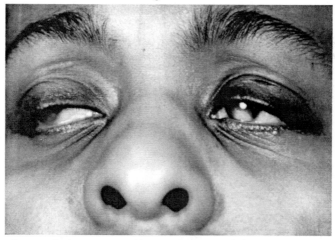

This photograph shows a stromal haze in both eyes of this male child due to his late-staged congenital syphilitic condition called interstitial keratitis (IK). Interstitial keratitis, which is an inflammation of the connective tissue structure of the cornea, usually affects both eyes, and can occur as a complication to congenital, or acquired, syphilis. IK usually occurs in children older than two years of age. Source PHIL

Diagnosis

Some health care providers can diagnose syphilis by examining material from a chancre (infectious sore) using a special microscope called a dark-field microscope. If syphilis bacteria are present in the sore, they will show up when observed through the microscope.

A blood test is another way to determine whether someone has syphilis. Shortly after infection occurs, the body produces syphilis antibodies that can be detected by an accurate, safe, and inexpensive blood test. A low level of antibodies will stay in the blood for months or years even after the disease has been successfully treated. Because untreated syphilis in a pregnant woman can infect and possibly kill her developing baby, every pregnant woman should have a blood test for syphilis.

Syphilis increases susceptibility to HIV

Genital sores (chancres) caused by syphilis make it easier to transmit and acquire HIV infection sexually. There is an estimated 2- to 5-fold increased risk of acquiring HIV infection when syphilis is present.

Ulcerative STDs that cause sores, ulcers, or breaks in the skin or mucous membranes, such as syphilis, disrupt barriers that provide protection against infections. The genital ulcers caused by syphilis can bleed easily, and when they come into contact with oral and rectal mucosa during sex, increase the infectiousness of and susceptibility to HIV. Having other STDs is also an important predictor for becoming HIV infected because STDs are a marker for behaviors associated with HIV transmission.

Treatment

Syphilis is easy to cure in its early stages. A single intramuscular injection of penicillin, an antibiotic, will cure a person who has had syphilis for less than a year. Additional doses are needed to treat someone who has had syphilis for longer than a year. For people who are allergic to penicillin, other antibiotics are available to treat syphilis. There are no home remedies or over-the-counter drugs that will cure syphilis. Treatment will kill the syphilis bacterium and prevent further damage, but it will not repair damage already done.

Because effective treatment is available, it is important that persons be screened for syphilis on an on-going basis if their sexual behaviors put them at risk for STDs.

Persons who receive syphilis treatment must abstain from sexual contact with new partners until the syphilis sores are completely healed. Persons with syphilis must notify their sex partners so that they also can be tested and receive treatment if necessary.

Having syphilis once does not protect a person from getting it again. Following successful treatment, people can still be susceptible to re-infection. Only laboratory tests can confirm whether someone has syphilis. Because syphilis sores can be hidden in the vagina, rectum, or mouth, it may not be obvious that a sex partner has syphilis. Talking with a health care provider will help to determine the need to be re-tested for syphilis after treatment has been received.

Prevention

The surest way to avoid transmission of sexually transmitted diseases, including syphilis, is to abstain from sexual contact or to be in a long-term mutually monogamous relationship with a partner who has been tested and is known to be uninfected.

Avoiding alcohol and drug use may also help prevent transmission of syphilis because these activities may lead to risky sexual behavior. It is important that sex partners talk to each other about their HIV status and history of other STDs so that preventive action can be taken.

Genital ulcer diseases, like syphilis, can occur in both male and female genital areas that are covered or protected by a latex condom, as well as in areas that are not covered. Correct and consistent use of latex condoms can reduce the risk of syphilis, as well as genital herpes and chancroid, only when the infected area or site of potential exposure is protected.

Condoms lubricated with spermicides (especially Nonoxynol-9 or N-9) are no more effective than other lubricated condoms in protecting against the transmission of STDs. Based on findings from several research studies, N-9 may itself cause genital lesions, providing a point of entry for HIV and other STDs. In June 2001, the CDC recommended that N-9 not be used as a microbicide or lubricant during anal intercourse. Transmission of a STD, including syphilis cannot be prevented by washing the genitals, urinating, and or douching after sex. Any unusual discharge, sore, or rash, particularly in the groin area, should be a signal to refrain from having sex and to see a doctor immediately.

The CDC's 2002 Sexually Transmitted Diseases Treatment Guidelines recommend that MSM who are at risk for STDs be tested for syphilis annually.

Sources

Centers for Disease Control and Prevention. Sexually transmitted diseases treatment guidelines 2002. MMWR 2002;51(no. RR-6).

http://www.cdc.gov/mmwr/PDF/RR/RR5106.pdf

Centers for Disease Control and Prevention. Sexually Transmitted Disease Surveillance, 2002. Atlanta, GA: U.S. Department of Health and Human Service, September 2003.

http://www.cdc.gov/std/stats02/toc2002.htm

K. Holmes, P. Mardh, P. Sparling et al (eds). Sexually Transmitted Diseases, 3rd Edition. New York: McGraw-Hill, 1999, chapters 33-37.

Centers for Disease Control and Prevention. HIV/STD Risks in Young Men Who Have Sex With Men Who Do Not Disclose Their Sexual Orientation – Six U.S. Cities, 1994 – 2000. MMWR 2003;52(05);81.
http://www.cdc.gov/mmwr/PDF/wk/mm5205.pdf

Centers for Disease Control and Prevention. Primary and Secondary Syphilis Among Men Who Have Sex With Men – New York City, 2001. MMWR 2002;51(38);853.

http://www.cdc.gov/mmwr/PDF/wk/mm5138.pdf

Centers for Disease Control and Prevention. Primary and Secondary Syphilis– United States,2000—2001.MMWR2002;51(43):971.

http://www.cdc.gov/mmwr/PDF/wk/mm5143.pdf

Centers for Disease Control and Prevention. Unrecognized HIV Infection, Risk Behaviors, and Perceptions of Risk Among Young Black Men Who Have Sex with Men — Six U.S. Cities, 1994 -1998. MMWR 2002;51(33);733.

http://www.cdc.gov/mmwr/PDF/wk/mm5133.pdf

Centers for Disease Control and Prevention. HIV Incidence Among Young Men Who Have Sex With Men– Seven U.S. Cities, 1994 – 2000. MMWR 2001;50(21);440.

http://www.cdc.gov/mmwr/PDF/wk/mm5021.pdf

Centers for Disease Control and Prevention. HIV and AIDS – United States, 1982-2000. MMWR 2001;50(21);430.

http://www.cdc.gov/mmwr/PDF/wk/mm5021.pdf

Centers for Disease Control and Prevention. Outbreak of Syphilis Among Men Who Have Sex With Men – Southern California, 2000. MMWR 2001;50(07);117.

http://www.cdc.gov/mmwr/preview/mmwrhtml/mm5007a2.htm

Centers for Disease Control and Prevention. Notice to Readers: CDC Statement on Study Results of Product Containing Nonoxynol-9. MMWR 2000;49(31);717.

http://www.cdc.gov/mmwr/preview/mmwrhtml/mm4931a4.htm

Centers for Disease Control and Prevention. STD Increases Among Gay and Bisexual Men. Reported at 2000 National STD Prevention Conference in Milwaukee, Wisconsin. December 2000.

http://www.cdc.gov/nchstp/dstd/Press_Releases/STDGay2000.htm

Centers for Disease Control and Prevention. Resurgent Bacterial Sexually Transmitted Disease Among Men Who Have Sex With Men – King County, Washington, MMWR 1999;48(35);773.

http://www.cdc.gov/mmwr/PDF/wk/mm4835.pdf

Centers for Disease Control and Prevention. HIV Prevention Through Early Detection and Treatment of Other Sexually Transmitted Diseases - United States Recommendations of the Advisory Committee for HIV and STD Prevention. MMWR 1998;47(RR12);1.

http://www.cdc.gov/mmwr/PDF/RR/RR4712.pdf

122

Trichomoniasis

Trichomoniasis is the most common curable STD in young, sexually active women. An estimated 7.4 million new cases occur each year in women and men.

Trichomoniasis affects both women and men, although symptoms are more common in women.

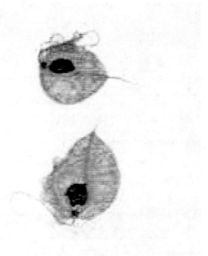

Photomicrograph of *Trichomonas vaginalis*

Trichomoniasis is caused by the single-celled protozoan parasite, Trichomonas vaginalis. The vagina is the most common site of infection in women, and the urethra (urine canal) is the most common site of infection in men. The parasite is sexually transmitted through penis-to-vagina intercourse or vulva-to-vulva (the genital area outside the vagina) contact with an infected partner. Women can acquire the disease from infected men or women, but men usually contract it only from infected women.

Symptoms

Most men with trichomoniasis do not have signs or symptoms; however, some men may temporarily have an irritation inside the penis, mild discharge, or slight burning after urination or ejaculation.

Some women have signs or symptoms of infection which include a frothy, yellow-green vaginal discharge with a strong odor. The infection also may cause discomfort during intercourse and urination, as well as irritation and itching of the female genital area. In rare cases, lower abdominal pain can occur. Symptoms usually appear in women within 5 to 28 days of exposure.

The genital inflammation caused by trichomoniasis can increase a woman's susceptibility to HIV infection if she is exposed to the virus. Having trichomoniasis may increase the chance that an HIV-infected woman passes HIV to her sex partner(s).

Trichomoniasis and Pregnancy

Pregnant women with trichomoniasis may have babies who are born early or with low birth weight (less than five pounds).

Diagnosis and Treatment

For both men and women, a health care provider must perform a physical examination and laboratory test to diagnose trichomoniasis. The parasite is harder to detect in men than in women. In women, a pelvic examination can reveal small red ulcerations (sores) on the vaginal wall or cervix.

Trichomoniasis can usually be cured with the prescription drug, metronidazole, given by mouth in a single dose. The symptoms of trichomoniasis in infected men may disappear within a few weeks without treatment. However, an infected man, even a man who has never had symptoms or whose symptoms have stopped, can continue to infect or re-infect a female partner until he has been treated. Therefore, both partners should be treated at the same time to eliminate the parasite. Persons being treated for trichomoniasis should avoid sex until they and their sex partners complete treatment and have no symptoms. Metronidazole can be used by pregnant women.

Having trichomoniasis once does not protect a person from getting it again. Following successful treatment, people can still be susceptible to re-infection.

124

Prevention

The surest way to avoid transmission of sexually transmitted diseases is to abstain from sexual contact, or to be in a long-term mutually monogamous relationship with a partner who has been tested and is known to be uninfected.

Latex male condoms, when used consistently and correctly, can reduce the risk of transmission of trichomoniasis.

Any genital symptom such as discharge or burning during urination or an unusual sore or rash should be a signal to stop having sex and to consult a health care provider immediately. A person diagnosed with trichomoniasis (or any other STD) should receive treatment and should notify all recent sex partners so that they can see a health care provider and be treated. This reduces the risk that the sex partners will develop complications from trichomoniasis and reduces the risk that the person with trichomoniasis will become re-infected. Sex should be stopped until the person with trichomoniasis and all of his or her recent partners complete treatment for trichomoniasis and have no symptoms.

Sources

Centers for Disease Control and Prevention. Sexually transmitted diseases treatment guidelines 2002. MMWR 2002;51(no. RR-6).

Krieger JN and Alderete JF. Trichomonas vaginalis and trichomoniasis. In: K. Holmes, P. Markh, P. Sparling et al (eds). Sexually Transmitted Diseases, 3rd Edition. New York: McGraw-Hill, 1999, 587-604.

Weinstock H, Berman S, Cates W. Sexually transmitted disease among American youth: Incidence and prevalence estimates, 2000. Perspectives on Sexual and Reproductive Health 2004; 36: 6-10.

Vaginal Infections and Vaginitis

Vaginal infections are frequent causes of distress and discomfort in adult women. The most common vaginal infections are bacterial vaginosis, trichomoniasis, and vulvovaginal candidiasis. Some vaginal infections are transmitted through sexual contact, but others such as candidiasis (yeast infections) are not.

Vaginal infections are often accompanied by vaginitis, which is an inflammation of the vagina characterized by discharge, irritation, and/or itching. The cause of vaginitis cannot be adequately determined solely on the basis of symptoms or a physical examination. Laboratory tests allowing microscopic evaluation of vaginal fluid are required for a correct diagnosis. A variety of effective drugs are available for treating vaginal infections and accompanying vaginitis.

Bacterial Vaginosis

Bacterial Vaginosis (BV) is the most common vaginal infection in women of childbearing age. In the United States, as many as 16 percent of pregnant women have BV.

Bacterial Vaginosis (BV) is the name of a condition in women where the normal balance of bacteria in the vagina is disrupted and replaced by an overgrowth of certain bacteria. It is sometimes accompanied by discharge, odor, pain, itching, or burning.

The cause of BV is not fully understood. BV is associated with an imbalance in the bacteria that are normally found in a woman's vagina. The vagina normally contains mostly "good" bacteria, and fewer "harmful" bacteria. BV develops when there is an increase in harmful bacteria.

Not much is known about how women get BV. There are many unanswered questions about the role that harmful bacteria play in

126

causing BV. Any woman can get BV. However, some activities or behaviors can upset the normal balance of bacteria in the vagina and put women at increased risk including:

- Having a new sex partner or multiple sex partners,
- Douching, and
- Using an intrauterine device (IUD) for contraception.

It is not clear what role sexual activity plays in the development of BV. Women do not get BV from toilet seats, bedding, swimming pools, or from touching objects around them. Women that have never had sexual intercourse are rarely affected.

Signs and Symptoms

Women with BV may have an abnormal vaginal discharge with an unpleasant odor. Some women report a strong fish-like odor, especially after intercourse. Discharge, if present, is usually white or gray; it can be thin. Women with BV may also have burning during urination or itching around the outside of the vagina, or both. Some women with BV report no signs or symptoms at all.

In most cases, BV causes no complications. But there are some serious risks from BV including:

- Having BV can increase a woman's susceptibility to HIV infection if she is exposed to the HIV virus.
- Having BV increases the chances that an HIV-infected woman can pass HIV to her sex partner.
- Having BV has been associated with an increase in the development of pelvic inflammatory disease (PID) following surgical procedures such as a hysterectomy or an abortion.
- Having BV while pregnant may put a woman at increased risk for some complications of pregnancy.
- BV can increase a woman's susceptibility to other STDs, such as Chlamydia and gonorrhea.

Effects on Pregnancy

Pregnant women with BV more often have babies who are born premature or with low birth weight (less than 5 pounds).

The bacteria that cause BV can sometimes infect the uterus (womb) and fallopian tubes (tubes that carry eggs from the ovaries to the uterus). This type of infection is called pelvic inflammatory disease (PID). PID can cause infertility or damage the fallopian tubes enough to increase the future risk of ectopic pregnancy and infertility. Ectopic pregnancy is a life-threatening condition in which a fertilized egg grows outside the uterus, usually in a fallopian tube which can rupture.

Diagnosis & Treatment

A health care provider must examine the vagina for signs of BV and perform laboratory tests on a sample of vaginal fluid to look for bacteria associated with BV.

Although BV will sometimes clear up without treatment, all women with symptoms of BV should be treated to avoid such complications as PID. Male partners generally do not need to be treated. However, BV may spread between female sex partners.

Treatment is especially important for pregnant women. All pregnant women who have ever had a premature delivery or low birth weight baby should be considered for a BV examination, regardless of symptoms, and should be treated if they have BV. All pregnant women who have symptoms of BV should be checked and treated.

Some physicians recommend that all women undergoing a hysterectomy or abortion be treated for BV prior to the procedure, regardless of symptoms, to reduce their risk of developing PID.

BV is treatable with antibiotics prescribed by a health care provider. Two different antibiotics are recommended as treatment for BV: metronidazole or clindamycin. Either can be used with non-pregnant or pregnant women, but the recommended dosages differ. Women with BV who are HIV-positive should receive the same treatment as those who are HIV-negative.

BV can recur after treatment.

Prevention

BV is not completely understood by scientists, and the best ways to prevent it are unknown. However, it is known that BV is associated with having a new sex partner or having multiple sex partners. It is seldom found in women who have never had intercourse.

The following basic prevention steps can help reduce the risk of upsetting the natural balance of bacteria in the vagina and developing BV:

- Be abstinent.
- Limit the number of sex partners.
- Do not douche.
- Use all of the medicine prescribed for treatment of BV, even if the signs and symptoms go away.

Sources

Centers for Disease Control and Prevention. Sexually transmitted diseases treatment guidelines 2002. MMWR 2002;51(no. RR-6

Hillier S and Holmes K. Bacterial vaginosis. In: K. Holmes, P. Sparling, P. Mardh et al (eds). Sexually Transmitted Diseases, 3rd Edition. New York: McGraw-Hill, 1999, 563-586

Vulvovaginal candidiasis (VVC)

Vulvovaginal candidiasis (VVC), sometimes referred to as candidal vaginitis, monilial infection, or vaginal yeast infection, is a common cause of vaginal irritation. It has been estimated that approximately 75 percent of all women will experience at least one episode of VVC during their lifetime. VVC is caused by an overabundance of yeast cells (primarily Candida albicans) that normally colonize in the vagina. Several factors are associated with increased rates of VVC in women, including pregnancy, uncontrolled diabetes mellitus, and the use of oral contraceptives or antibiotics. Other factors that may increase the incidence of VVC include the use of douches, perfumed feminine hygiene sprays, topical antimicrobial agents, and tight, poorly ventilated clothing and underwear. There is no direct evidence that VVC is transmitted by sexual intercourse.

Symptoms.

Most frequent symptoms of VVC in women are itching, burning, and irritation of the vagina. Painful urination and/or intercourse are common. Abnormal vaginal discharge is not always present and may be minimal. The discharge is typically described as cottage cheese-like in nature, although it may vary from watery to thick in consistency. Most male partners of women with VVC do not experience symptoms of the infection, though a transient rash and burning sensation of the penis have been reported after intercourse without condoms.

Diagnosis.

As few specific signs and symptoms are usually present, VVC cannot be diagnosed by the patient's history and physical examination. VVC is usually diagnosed through microscopic examination of vaginal secretions for evidence of yeast forms.

Treatment.

Various antifungal vaginal creams are available to treat VVC. Some antifungal creams (miconazole and clotrimazole) are available over the counter for use in the vagina; however, because BV, trichomoniasis, and VVC are difficult to distinguish on the basis of symptoms alone, a woman with vaginal symptoms should see a physician for an accurate diagnosis before using these products. Other products available over the counter contain antihistamines or topical anesthetics that only mask the symptoms and do not treat the underlying problem. Women who have chronic or recurring VVC may need to be treated for extended periods of time and may be given oral antifungal drugs. They should work with their physicians to determine possible underlying causes of their chronic yeast infections. Because there is no evidence for sexual transmission of VVC, routine treatment of male partners is unlikely to reduce recurrence.

Other Causes of Vaginitis

Although most vaginal infections in women are due to bacterial vaginosis, trichomoniasis, and vulvovaginal candidiasis, it is clear that there are other causes. These causes may include allergic and irritative factors or other STDs. Noninfectious allergic symptoms can be caused by spermicides, vaginal hygiene products, detergents, and fabric softeners. Cervical infections are also often associated with abnormal vaginal discharge, but these infections can be distinguished from true vaginal infections by appropriate tests. Finally, in uninfected women, vaginal discharge may be present during ovulation and may become so heavy that it raises concern.

Research is under way to determine the factors that promote the growth and disease-causing potential of vaginal microbes. Vaginitis is no longer considered merely a benign annoyance, and scientists are working to clarify its role in such conditions as pelvic inflammatory disease and pregnancy-related complications.

HIV Infection and AIDS

AIDS (acquired immunodeficiency syndrome) was first reported in the United States in 1981 and has since become a major worldwide epidemic. AIDS is caused by HIV (human immunodeficiency virus). By killing or damaging cells of the body's immune system, HIV progressively destroys the body's ability to fight infections and certain cancers. People diagnosed with AIDS may get life-threatening diseases called opportunistic infections, which are caused by microbes such as viruses or bacteria that usually do not make healthy people sick.

More than 900,000 cases of AIDS have been reported in the United States since 1981. As many as 950,000 Americans may be infected with HIV, one-quarter of whom are unaware of their infection. The epidemic is growing most rapidly among minority populations and is a leading killer of African-American males ages 25 to 44. According to the Centers for Disease Control and Prevention (CDC), AIDS affects nearly seven times more African Americans and three times more Hispanics than whites. In recent years, an increasing number of African-American women and children are being affected by HIV/AIDS. In 2003, two-thirds of U.S. AIDS cases in both women and children were among African-Americans.

TRANSMISSION

Research has revealed a great deal of valuable medical, scientific, and public health information about the human immunodeficiency virus (HIV) and acquired immunodeficiency syndrome (AIDS). The ways in which HIV can be transmitted have been clearly identified. Unfortunately, false information or statements that are not supported by scientific findings continue to be shared widely through the Internet or popular press.

HIV is spread most commonly by having unprotected sex with an infected partner. The virus can enter the body through the lining of the vagina, vulva, penis, rectum, or mouth during sex. HIV is spread by sexual contact with an infected person, by sharing needles and/or syringes (primarily for drug injection) with someone who is infected, or, less commonly (and now very rarely in countries where blood is screened for HIV antibodies), through transfusions of infected blood or blood clotting factors. Babies born to HIV-infected women may become infected before or during birth or through breast-feeding after birth.

Some people fear that HIV might be transmitted in other ways; however, no scientific evidence to support any of these fears has been found. If HIV were being transmitted through other routes (such as through air, water, or insects), the pattern of reported AIDS cases would be much different from what has been observed. For example, if mosquitoes could transmit HIV infection, many more young children and preadolescents would have been diagnosed with AIDS.

All reported cases suggesting new or potentially unknown routes of transmission are thoroughly investigated by state and local health departments with the assistance, guidance, and laboratory support from CDC. *No additional routes of transmission have been recorded*, despite a national sentinel system designed to detect just such an occurrence.

Risky behavior

HIV can infect anyone who practices risky behaviors such as

- Sharing drug needles or syringes
- Having sexual contact, including oral, with an infected person without using a condom
- Having sexual contact with someone whose HIV status is unknown

---

Infected blood

HIV also is spread through contact with infected blood. Before donated blood was screened for evidence of HIV infection and before heat-treating techniques to destroy HIV in blood products were introduced, HIV was transmitted through transfusions of contaminated blood or blood components. Today, because of blood screening and heat treatment, the risk of getting HIV from such transfusions is extremely small.

Contaminated needles

HIV is frequently spread among injection drug users by the sharing of needles or syringes contaminated with very small quantities of blood from someone infected with the virus.

It is rare, however, for a patient to give HIV to a health care worker or vice-versa by accidental sticks with contaminated needles or other medical instruments.

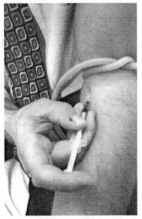

In the health care setting, workers have been infected with HIV after being stuck with needles containing HIV-infected blood or, less frequently, after infected blood gets into a worker's open cut or a mucous membrane (for example, the eyes or inside of the nose). There has been only one instance of patients being infected by a health care worker in the United States; this involved HIV transmission from one infected dentist to six patients. Investigations have been completed involving more than 22,000 patients of 63 HIV-infected physicians, surgeons, and dentists, and no other cases of this type of transmission have been identified in the United States.

Mother to child

Women can transmit HIV to their babies during pregnancy or birth. Approximately one-quarter to one-third of all untreated pregnant women infected with HIV will pass the infection to their babies. HIV also can be spread to babies through the breast milk of mothers infected with the virus. If the mother takes certain drugs during pregnancy, she can significantly reduce the chances that her baby will get infected with HIV. If health care providers treat HIV-infected pregnant women and deliver their babies by cesarean section, the chances of the baby being infected can be reduced to a rate of 1 percent. HIV infection of newborns has been almost eradicated in the United States due to appropriate treatment.

A study sponsored by the National Institute of Allergy and Infectious Diseases (NIAID) in Uganda found a highly effective and safe drug for preventing transmission of HIV from an infected mother to her newborn. Independent studies have also confirmed this finding. This regimen is more affordable and practical than any other examined to date. Results from the study show that a single oral dose of the antiretroviral drug nevirapine (NVP) given to an HIV-infected woman in labor and another to her baby within 3 days of birth reduces the transmission rate of HIV by half compared with a similar short course of AZT (Azidothymidine).

Sexually transmitted infections

If you have a sexually transmitted infection (STI) such as syphilis, genital herpes, chlamydial infection, gonorrhea, or bacterial vaginosis appears, you may be more susceptible to getting HIV infection during sex with infected partners.

Casual contact

Studies of families of HIV-infected people have shown clearly that HIV is not spread through casual contact such as the sharing of food utensils, towels and bedding, swimming pools, telephones, or toilet seats.

HIV is not spread by biting insects such as mosquitoes or bedbugs.

HIV in the Environment

Scientists and medical authorities agree that HIV does not survive well in the environment, making the possibility of environmental transmission remote. HIV is found in varying concentrations or amounts in blood, semen, vaginal fluid, breast milk, saliva, and tears. To obtain data on the survival of HIV, laboratory studies have required the use of artificially high concentrations of laboratory-grown virus. Although these unnatural concentrations of HIV can be kept alive for days or even weeks under precisely controlled and limited laboratory conditions, CDC studies have shown that drying of even these high concentrations of HIV reduces the amount of infectious virus by 90 to 99 percent within several hours. Since the HIV concentrations used in laboratory studies are much higher than those actually found in blood or other specimens, drying of HIV-infected human blood or other body fluids reduces the theoretical risk of environmental transmission to that which has been observed--essentially zero. Incorrect interpretations of conclusions drawn from laboratory studies have unnecessarily alarmed some people.

Results from laboratory studies should not be used to assess specific personal risk of infection because (1) the amount of virus studied is not found in human specimens or elsewhere in nature, and (2) no one has been identified as infected with HIV due to contact with an environmental surface. Additionally, HIV is unable to reproduce outside its living host (unlike many bacteria or fungi, which may do so under suitable conditions), except under laboratory conditions, therefore, it does not spread or maintain infectiousness outside its host.

Households

Although HIV has been transmitted between family members in a household setting, this type of transmission is very rare. These transmissions are believed to have resulted from contact between skin or mucous membranes and infected blood. To prevent even such rare occurrences, precautions, as described in previously published guidelines, should be taken in all settings "including the home" to prevent exposures to the blood of persons who are HIV infected, at risk for HIV infection, or whose infection and risk status are unknown. For example,

- Gloves should be worn during contact with blood or other body fluids that could possibly contain visible blood, such as urine, feces, or vomit.

- Cuts, sores, or breaks on both the care giver's and patient's exposed skin should be covered with bandages.

137

- Hands and other parts of the body should be washed immediately after contact with blood or other body fluids, and surfaces soiled with blood should be disinfected appropriately.

- Practices that increase the likelihood of blood contact, such as sharing of razors and toothbrushes, should be avoided.

- Needles and other sharp instruments should be used only when medically necessary and handled according to recommendations for health-care settings. (Do not put caps back on needles by hand or remove needles from syringes. Dispose of needles in puncture-proof containers

Businesses and Other Settings

There is no known risk of HIV transmission to co-workers, clients, or consumers from contact in industries such as food-service establishments (see information on survival of HIV in the environment). Food-service workers known to be infected with HIV need not be restricted from work unless they have other infections or illnesses (such as diarrhea or hepatitis A) for which any food-service worker, regardless of HIV infection status, should be restricted. CDC recommends that all food-service workers follow recommended standards and practices of good personal hygiene and food sanitation.

In 1985, CDC issued routine precautions that all personal-service workers (such as hairdressers, barbers, cosmetologists, and massage therapists) should follow, even though there is no evidence of transmission from a personal-service worker to a client or vice versa. Instruments that are intended to penetrate the skin (such as tattooing and acupuncture needles, ear piercing devices) should be used once and disposed of or thoroughly cleaned and sterilized. Instruments not intended to penetrate the skin but which may become contaminated with blood (for example, razors) should be used for only one client and disposed of or thoroughly cleaned and disinfected after each use. Personal-service workers can use the same cleaning procedures that are recommended for health care institutions.

CDC knows of no instances of HIV transmission through tattooing or body piercing, although hepatitis B virus has been transmitted during some of these practices. One case of HIV transmission from acupuncture has been documented. Body piercing (other than ear piercing) is relatively new in the United States, and the medical complications for body piercing appear to be greater than for tattoos. Healing of piercings generally will take weeks, and sometimes even months, and the pierced tissue could conceivably be abraded (torn or cut) or inflamed even after healing. Therefore, a theoretical HIV transmission risk does exist if the unhealed or abraded tissues come into contact with an infected person's blood or other infectious body fluid. Additionally, HIV could be transmitted if instruments contaminated with blood are not sterilized or disinfected between clients.

Saliva, Tears, and Sweat

Although researchers have found HIV in the saliva of infected people, there is no evidence that the virus is spread by contact with saliva. It is important to understand that finding a small amount of HIV in a body fluid does not necessarily mean that HIV can be *transmitted* by that body fluid. Laboratory studies reveal that saliva has natural properties that limit the power of HIV to infect, and the amount of virus in saliva appears to be very low. Research studies of people infected with HIV have found no evidence that the virus is spread to others through saliva by kissing. The lining of the mouth, however, can be infected by HIV, and instances of HIV transmission through oral intercourse have been reported.

HIV has *not* been recovered from the sweat of HIV-infected persons.

Scientists have found no evidence that HIV is spread through sweat, tears, urine, or feces.

Kissing

Casual contact through closed-mouth or "social" kissing is not a risk for transmission of HIV. Because of the potential for contact with blood during "French" or open-mouth kissing, CDC recommends against engaging in this activity with a person known to be infected. However, the risk of acquiring HIV during open-mouth kissing is believed to be very low. CDC has investigated only one case of HIV infection that may be attributed to contact with blood during open-mouth kissing.

Biting

In 1997, CDC published findings from a state health department investigation of an incident that suggested blood-to-blood transmission of HIV by a human bite. There have been other reports in the medical literature in which HIV appeared to have been transmitted by a bite. Severe trauma with extensive tissue tearing and damage and presence of blood were reported in each of these instances. Biting is not a common way of transmitting HIV. In fact, there are numerous reports of bites that did *not* result in HIV infection.

Insects

From the onset of the HIV epidemic, there has been concern about transmission of the virus by biting and bloodsucking insects. However, studies conducted by researchers at CDC and elsewhere have shown no evidence of HIV transmission through insects--even in areas where there are many cases of AIDS and large populations of insects such as mosquitoes. Lack of such outbreaks, despite intense efforts to detect them, supports the conclusion that HIV is not transmitted by insects.

The results of experiments and observations of insect biting behavior indicate that when an insect bites a person, it does not inject its own or a previously bitten person's or animal's blood into the next person bitten. Rather, it injects saliva, which acts as a lubricant or anticoagulant so the insect can feed efficiently. Such diseases as yellow fever and malaria are transmitted through the saliva of specific species of mosquitoes. However, HIV lives for only a short time inside an insect and, unlike organisms that are transmitted via insect bites, HIV does not reproduce (and does not survive) in insects. Thus, even if the virus enters a mosquito or another sucking or biting insect, the insect does not become infected and cannot transmit HIV to the next human it feeds on or bites. HIV is not found in insect feces.

There is also no reason to fear that a biting or bloodsucking insect, such as a mosquito, could transmit HIV from one person to another through HIV-infected blood left on its mouth parts. Two factors serve to explain why this is so--first, infected people do not have constant, high levels of HIV in their bloodstreams and, second, insect mouth parts do not retain large amounts of blood on their surfaces. Further, scientists who study insects have determined that biting insects normally do not travel from one person to the next immediately after ingesting blood. Rather, they fly to a resting place to digest this blood meal.

EARLY SYMPTOMS OF HIV INFECTION

If you are like many people, you will not have any symptoms when you first become infected with HIV. You may, however, have a flu-like illness within a month or two after exposure to the virus. This illness may include

- Fever
- Headache
- Tiredness
- Enlarged lymph nodes (glands of the immune system easily felt in the neck and groin)

These symptoms usually disappear within a week to a month and are often mistaken for those of another viral infection. During this period, people are very infectious, and HIV is present in large quantities in genital fluids.

More persistent or severe symptoms may not appear for 10 years or more after HIV first enters the body in adults, or within 2 years in children born with HIV infection. This period of "asymptomatic" infection varies greatly in each individual. Some people may begin to have symptoms within a few months, while others may be symptom-free for more than 10 years.

Even during the asymptomatic period, the virus is actively multiplying, infecting, and killing cells of the immune system. The virus can also hide within infected cells and lay dormant. The most obvious effect of HIV infection is a decline in the number of CD4 positive T (CD4+) cells found in the blood-the immune system's key infection fighters. The virus slowly disables or destroys these cells without causing symptoms.

Progression of HIV Infection

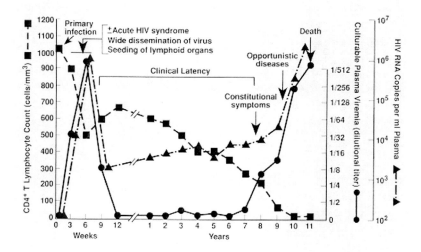

As the immune system worsens, a variety of complications start to take over. For many people, the first signs of infection are large lymph nodes or "swollen glands" that may be enlarged for more than 3 months. Other symptoms often experienced months to years before the onset of AIDS include

- Lack of energy
- Weight loss

- Frequent fevers and sweats
- Persistent or frequent yeast infections (oral or vaginal)
- Persistent skin rashes or flaky skin
- Pelvic inflammatory disease in women that does not respond to treatment
- Short-term memory loss

Some people develop frequent and severe herpes infections that cause mouth, genital, or anal sores, or a painful nerve disease called shingles. Children may grow slowly or be sick a lot.

WHAT IS AIDS?

The term AIDS applies to the most advanced stages of HIV infection. CDC developed official criteria for the definition of AIDS and is responsible for tracking the spread of AIDS in the United States.

CDC's definition of AIDS includes all HIV-infected people who have fewer than 200 CD4+ T cells per cubic millimeter of blood. (Healthy adults usually have CD4+ T-cell counts of 1,000 or more.) In addition, the definition includes 26 clinical conditions that affect people with advanced HIV disease. Most of these conditions are opportunistic infections that generally do not affect healthy people. In people with AIDS, these infections are often severe and sometimes fatal because the immune system is so ravaged by HIV that the body cannot fight off certain bacteria, viruses, fungi, parasites, and other microbes.

Symptoms of opportunistic infections common in people with AIDS include

- Coughing and shortness of breath
- Seizures and lack of coordination
- Difficult or painful swallowing
- Mental symptoms such as confusion and forgetfulness

- Severe and persistent diarrhea
- Fever
- Vision loss
- Nausea, abdominal cramps, and vomiting
- Weight loss and extreme fatigue
- Severe headaches
- Coma

Children with AIDS may get the same opportunistic infections as do adults with the disease. In addition, they also have severe forms of the typically common childhood bacterial infections, such as conjunctivitis (pink eye), ear infections, and tonsillitis.

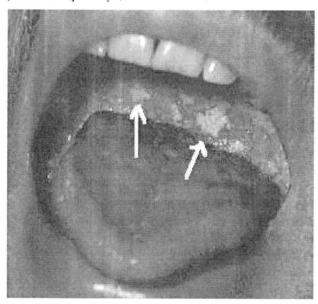

Persistent incidence of Thrush, a yeast infection in the mouth, often results from HIV weakening body defenses. Photo courtesy of Tri D. Do at the Boston University Medical School

People with AIDS are also particularly prone to developing various cancers, especially those caused by viruses such as Kaposi's sarcoma and cervical cancer, or cancers of the immune system known as lymphomas. These cancers are usually more aggressive and difficult to treat in people with AIDS. Signs of Kaposi's sarcoma in light-skinned people are round brown, reddish, or purple spots that develop in the skin or in the mouth. In dark-skinned people, the spots are more pigmented.

During the course of HIV infection, most people experience a gradual decline in the number of CD4+ T cells, although some may have abrupt and dramatic drops in their CD4+ T-cell counts. A person with CD4+ T cells above 200 may experience some of the early symptoms of HIV disease. Others may have no symptoms even though their CD4+ T-cell count is below 200.

Many people are so debilitated by the symptoms of AIDS that they cannot hold a steady job or do household chores. Other people with AIDS may experience phases of intense life-threatening illness followed by phases in which they function normally.

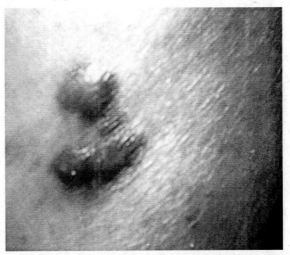

This brown cutaneous nodule represents a Kaposi's sarcoma lesion commonly found in patients with AIDS. Before the onset of the AIDS pandemic, Kaposi's sarcoma was an uncommon malignancy found mainly amongst Mediterranean men, African children and Ashkenazi Jews, but became the most common neoplasm found in those with AIDS. Source PHIL

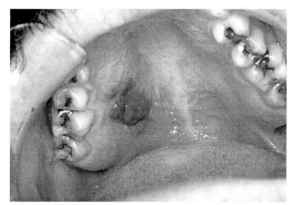

This HIV patient presented with intraoral Kaposi's sarcoma of the hard palate secondary to his AIDS infection. In approximately 7.5-10 percent of AIDS patients display signs of oral Kaposi's sarcoma, and can range in appearance from a small asymptomatic growths that are flat purple-red in color, to larger nodular growths. Source PHIL

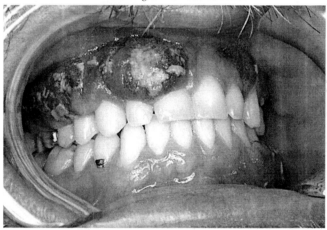

This HIV-positive patient presented with an intraoral Kaposi's sarcoma lesion with an overlying candidiasis infection. Initially, the KS lesions are flattened and red, but as they age they become raised, and darker, tending to purple. Source PHIL.

146

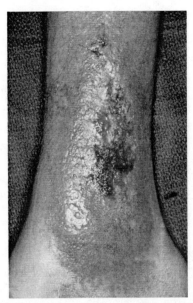

This lesion turned out to be Kaposi's sarcoma of the distal leg, but initially appeared to be a stasis dermatitis ulcer. In more recent years, the vast majority of cases of Kaposi's sarcoma are found in patients with AIDS. The most common site for KS is on the skin but it may also affect internal organs, particularly the lymph nodes, the lungs and digestive system. Source PHIL

A small number of people first infected with HIV 10 or more years ago have not developed symptoms of AIDS. Scientists are trying to determine what factors may account for their lack of progression to AIDS, such as

- Whether their immune systems have particular characteristics
- Whether they were infected with a less aggressive strain of the virus
- If their genes may protect them from the effects of HIV

Scientists hope that understanding the body's natural method of controlling infection may lead to ideas for protective HIV vaccines and use of vaccines to prevent the disease from progressing.

DIAGNOSIS

Because early HIV infection often causes no symptoms, your health care provider usually can diagnose it by testing your blood for the presence of antibodies (disease-fighting proteins) to HIV. HIV antibodies generally do not reach noticeable levels in the blood for 1 to 3 months following infection. It may take the antibodies as long as 6 months to be produced in quantities large enough to show up in standard blood tests. Hence, to determine whether you have been recently infected (acute infection), your health care provider can screen you for the presence of HIV genetic material. Direct screening of HIV is extremely critical in order to prevent transmission of HIV from recently infected individuals.

If you have been exposed to the virus, you should get an HIV test as soon as you are likely to develop antibodies to the virus-within 6 weeks to 12 months after possible exposure to the virus. By getting tested early, if infected, you can discuss with your health care provider when you should start treatment to help your immune system combat HIV and help prevent the emergence of certain opportunistic infections (see section on treatment below). Early testing also alerts you to avoid high-risk behaviors that could spread the virus to others.

Most health care providers can do HIV testing and will usually offer you counseling at the same time. Of course, you can be tested anonymously at many sites if you are concerned about confidentiality.

Health care providers diagnose HIV infection by using two different types of antibody tests: ELISA and Western Blot. If you are highly likely to be infected with HIV but have been tested negative for both tests, your health care provider may request additional tests. You also may be told to repeat antibody testing at a later date, when antibodies to HIV are more likely to have developed.

Babies born to mothers infected with HIV may or may not be infected with the virus, but all carry their mothers' antibodies to HIV for several months. If these babies lack symptoms, a doctor

148

cannot make a definitive diagnosis of HIV infection using standard antibody. Health care providers are using new technologies to detect HIV to more accurately determine HIV infection in infants between ages 3 months and 15 months. They are evaluating a number of blood tests to determine which ones are best for diagnosing HIV infection in babies younger than 3 months.

TREATMENT

When AIDS first surfaced in the United States, there were no medicines to combat the underlying immune deficiency and few treatments existed for the opportunistic diseases that resulted. Researchers, however, have developed drugs to fight both HIV infection and its associated infections and cancers.

Treatment of HIV infection

The Food and Drug Administration (FDA) has approved a number of drugs for treating HIV infection. The first group of drugs used to treat HIV infection, called nucleoside reverse transcriptase (RT) inhibitors, interrupts an early stage of the virus making copies of itself. These drugs may slow the spread of HIV in the body and delay the start of opportunistic infections. This class of drugs, called nucleoside analogs, includes

- AZT (Azidothymidine)
- ddC (zalcitabine)
- ddI (dideoxyinosine)
- d4T (stavudine)
- 3TC (lamivudine)
- Abacavir (ziagen)
- Tenofovir (viread)
- Emtriva (emtricitabine)

Health care providers can prescribe non-nucleoside reverse transcriptase inhibitors (NNRTIs), such as

- Delavridine (Rescriptor)
- Nevirapine (Viramune)

- Efravirenz (Sustiva) (in combination with other anti-retroviral drugs)

FDA also has approved a second class of drugs for treating HIV infection. These drugs, called protease inhibitors, interrupt the virus from making copies of itself at a later step in its life cycle. They include

- Ritonavir (Norvir)
- Saquinivir (Invirase)
- Indinavir (Crixivan)
- Amprenivir (Agenerase)
- Nelfinavir (Viracept)
- Lopinavir (Kaletra)
- Atazanavir (Reyataz)
- Fosamprenavir (Lexiva)

FDA also has introduced a third new class of drugs, known at fusion inhibitors, to treat HIV infection. Fuzeon (enfuvirtide or T-20), the first approved fusion inhibitor, works by interfering with HIV-1's ability to enter into cells by blocking the merging of the virus with the cell membranes. This inhibition blocks HIV's ability to enter and infect the human immune cells. Fuzeon is designed for use in combination with other anti-HIV treatment. It reduces the level of HIV infection in the blood and may be active against HIV that has become resistant to current antiviral treatment schedules.

Because HIV can become resistant to any of these drugs, health care providers must use a combination treatment to effectively suppress the virus. When multiple drugs (three or more) are used in combination, it is referred to as highly active antiretroviral therapy, or HAART, and can be used by people who are newly infected with HIV as well as people with AIDS.

Researchers have credited HAART as being a major factor in significantly reducing the number of deaths from AIDS in this country. While HAART is not a cure for AIDS, it has greatly improved the health of many people with AIDS and it reduces the amount of virus circulating in the blood to nearly undetectable levels. Researchers, however, have shown that HIV remains present in hiding places, such as the lymph nodes, brain, testes, and retina of the eye, even in people who have been treated.

Side effects

Despite the beneficial effects of HAART, there are side effects associated with the use of antiviral drugs that can be severe. Some of the nucleoside RT inhibitors may cause a decrease of red or white blood cells, especially when taken in the later stages of the disease. Some may also cause inflammation of the pancreas and painful nerve damage. There have been reports of complications and other severe reactions, including death, to some of the antiretroviral nucleoside analogs when used alone or in combination. Therefore, health care experts recommend that you be routinely seen and followed by your health care provider if you are on antiretroviral therapy.

The most common side effects associated with protease inhibitors include nausea, diarrhea, and other gastrointestinal symptoms. In addition, protease inhibitors can interact with other drugs resulting in serious side effects. Fuzeon may also cause severe allergic reactions such as pneumonia, trouble breathing, chills and fever, skin rash, blood in urine, vomiting, and low blood pressure. Local skin reactions are also possible since it is given as an injection underneath the skin.

If you are taking HIV drugs, you should contact your health care provider immediately if you have any of these symptoms.

Treatment of Opportunistic infections

A number of available drugs help treat opportunistic infections. These drugs include

- Foscarnet and ganciclovir to treat CMV (cytomegalovirus) eye infections
- Fluconazole to treat yeast and other fungal infections

- TMP/SMX (trimethoprim/sulfamethoxazole) or pentamidine to treat PCP (Pneumocystis carinii pneumonia)

Cancers

Health care providers use radiation, chemotherapy, or injections of alpha interferon-a genetically engineered protein that occurs naturally in the human body-to treat Kaposi's sarcoma or other cancers associated with HIV infection.

PREVENTION

Because no vaccine for HIV is available, the only way to prevent infection by the virus is to avoid behaviors that put you at risk of infection, such as sharing needles and having unprotected sex.

Many people infected with HIV have no symptoms. Therefore, there is no way of knowing with certainty whether your sexual partner is infected unless he or she has repeatedly tested negative for the virus and has not engaged in any risky behavior. You should either abstain from having sex or use male latex condoms or female polyurethane condoms, which may offer partial protection, during oral, anal, or vaginal sex. Only water-based lubricants should be used with male latex condoms.

Although some laboratory evidence shows that spermicides can kill HIV, researchers have not found that these products can prevent you from getting HIV.

Effectiveness of Condoms

Condoms are classified as medical devices and are regulated by the Food and Drug Administration (FDA). Condom manufacturers in the United States test each latex condom for defects, including holes, before it is packaged. The proper and consistent use of latex or polyurethane (a type of plastic) condoms when engaging in sexual intercourse--vaginal, anal, or oral--can greatly reduce a person's risk of acquiring or transmitting sexually transmitted diseases, including HIV infection.

There are many different types and brands of condoms available--however, only latex or polyurethane condoms provide a highly effective mechanical barrier to HIV. In laboratories, viruses occasionally have been shown to pass through natural membrane ("skin" or lambskin) condoms, which may contain natural pores and are therefore not recommended for disease prevention (they are documented to be effective for contraception). Women may wish to consider using the female condom when a male condom cannot be used.

For condoms to provide maximum protection, they must be used *consistently* (every time) and *correctly*. Several studies of correct and consistent condom use clearly show that latex condom breakage rates in this country are less than 2 percent. Even when condoms do break, one study showed that more than half of such breaks occurred prior to ejaculation.

When condoms are used reliably, they have been shown to prevent pregnancy up to 98 percent of the time among couples using them as their only method of contraception. Similarly, numerous studies among sexually active people have demonstrated that a properly used latex condom provides a high degree of protection against a variety of sexually transmitted diseases, including HIV infection.

RESEARCH

NIAID-supported investigators are conducting an abundance of research on all areas of HIV infection, including developing and testing preventive HIV vaccines and new treatments for HIV infection and AIDS-associated opportunistic infections. Researchers also are investigating exactly how HIV damages the immune system. This research is identifying new and more effective targets for drugs and vaccines. NIAID-supported investigators also continue to trace how the disease progresses in different people.

Scientists are investigating and testing chemical barriers, such as topical microbicides, that people can use in the vagina or in the rectum during sex to prevent HIV transmission. They also are looking at other ways to prevent transmission, such as controlling STIs and modifying personal behavior, as well as ways to prevent transmission from mother to child.

How HIV Causes AIDS

A significant component of the research effort of the National Institute of Allergy and Infectious Diseases (NIAID) is devoted to the pathogenesis of HIV (human immunodeficiency virus) disease. Studies on pathogenesis address the complex mechanisms that result in the destruction of the immune system of an HIV-infected person. A detailed understanding of HIV and how it establishes infection and causes AIDS (acquired immunodeficiency syndrome) is crucial to identifying and developing effective drugs and vaccines to fight HIV and AIDS. This fact sheet summarizes the state of knowledge in this area.

(Scientific terms printed in bold-faced type are defined in the Glossary at the end of this document.)

OVERVIEW

Untreated HIV disease is characterized by a gradual deterioration of immune function. Most notably, crucial immune cells called CD4 positive (CD4+) T cells are disabled and killed during the typical course of infection. These cells, sometimes called "T-helper cells," play a central role in the immune response, signaling other cells in the immune system to perform their special functions.

A healthy, uninfected person usually has 800 to 1,200 CD4+ T cells per cubic millimeter (mm3) of blood. During untreated HIV infection, the number of these cells in a person's blood progressively declines. When the CD4+ T cell count falls below 200/mm3, a person becomes particularly vulnerable to the opportunistic infections and cancers that typify AIDS, the end stage of HIV disease. People with AIDS often suffer infections of the lungs, intestinal tract, brain, eyes, and other organs, as well as debilitating weight loss, diarrhea, neurologic conditions, and cancers such as Kaposi's sarcoma and certain types of lymphomas.

Most scientists think that HIV causes AIDS by directly inducing the death of CD4+ T cells or interfering with their normal function, and by triggering other events that weaken a person's

154

immune function. For example, the network of signaling molecules that normally regulates a person's immune response is disrupted during HIV disease, impairing a person's ability to fight other infections. The HIV-mediated destruction of the lymph nodes and related immunologic organs also plays a major role in causing the immunosuppression seen in people with AIDS. Immunosuppression by HIV is confirmed by the fact that medicines, which interfere with the HIV lifecycle, preserve CD4+ T cells and immune function as well as delay clinical illness.

SCOPE OF THE HIV EPIDEMIC

Although HIV was first identified in 1983, studies of previously stored blood samples indicate that the virus entered the U.S. population sometime in the late 1970s. In the United States, 886,575 cases of AIDS, and 501,669 deaths among people with AIDS had been reported to the Centers for Disease Control and Prevention (CDC) by the end of 2002. Approximately 40,000 new HIV infections occur each year in the United States, 70 percent of them among men and 30 percent among women. Of the new infections, approximately 40 percent are from male-to-male contact, 30 percent from heterosexual contact, and 25 percent from injection drug use. Minority groups in the United States have also been disproportionately affected by the epidemic.

Worldwide, an estimated 38 million people were living with HIV/AIDS as of December 2003, according to the Joint United Nations Programme on HIV/AIDS (UNAIDS) . Through 2003, cumulative AIDS-associated deaths worldwide numbered more than 20 million. Globally, approximately 5 million new HIV infections and approximately 3 million AIDS-related deaths, including an estimated 490,000 children under 15 years old, occurred in the year 2003 alone.

HIV IS A RETROVIRUS

HIV belongs to a class of viruses called retroviruses . Retroviruses are RNA (ribonucleic acid) viruses, and in order to replicate (duplicate). they must make a DNA (deoxyribonucleic acid) copy of their RNA. It is the DNA genes that allow the virus to replicate.

Like all viruses, HIV can replicate only inside cells, commandeering the cell's machinery to reproduce. Only HIV and other retroviruses, however, once inside a cell, use an enzyme called reverse transcriptase to convert their RNA into DNA, which can be incorporated into the host cell's genes.

Slow viruses

HIV belongs to a subgroup of retroviruses known as lentiviruses , or "slow" viruses. The course of infection with these viruses is characterized by a long interval between initial infection and the onset of serious symptoms.

Other lentiviruses infect nonhuman species. For example, the feline immunodeficiency virus (FIV) infects cats and the simian immunodeficiency virus (SIV) infects monkeys and other nonhuman primates. Like HIV in humans, these animal viruses primarily infect immune system cells, often causing immune deficiency and AIDS-like symptoms. These viruses and their hosts have provided researchers with useful, albeit imperfect, models of the HIV disease process in people.

STRUCTURE OF HIV

The viral envelope

HIV has a diameter of 1/10,000 of a millimeter and is spherical in shape. The outer coat of the virus, known as the viral envelope, is composed of two layers of fatty molecules called lipids, taken from the membrane of a human cell when a newly formed virus particle buds from the cell. Evidence from NIAID-supported research indicates that HIV may enter and exit cells through special areas of the cell membrane known as "lipid rafts." These rafts are high in cholesterol and glycolipids and may provide a new target for blocking HIV.

Organization of the HIV-1 Virion

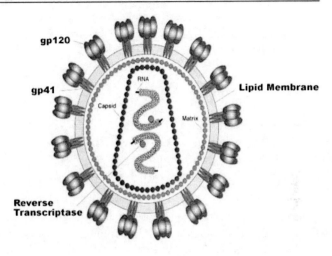

Embedded in the viral envelope are proteins from the host cell, as well as 72 copies (on average) of a complex HIV protein (frequently called "spikes") that protrudes through the surface of the virus particle (virion). This protein, known as Env, consists of a cap made of three molecules called glycoprotein (gp) 120, and a stem consisting of three gp41 molecules that anchor the structure in the viral envelope. Much of the research to develop a vaccine against HIV has focused on these envelope proteins.

The viral core

Within the envelope of a mature HIV particle is a bullet-shaped core or capsid, made of 2,000 copies of another viral protein, p24. The capsid surrounds two single strands of HIV RNA, each of which has a copy of the virus's nine genes. Three of these genes, gag, pol, and env , contain information needed to make structural proteins for new virus particles. The env gene, for example, codes for a protein called gp160 that is broken down by a viral enzyme to form gp120 and gp41, the components of Env.

Six regulatory genes, tat, rev, nef, vif, vpr, and vpu, contain information necessary to produce proteins that control the ability of

HIV to infect a cell, produce new copies of virus, or cause disease. The protein encoded by nef, for instance, appears necessary for the virus to replicate efficiently, and the vpu-encoded protein influences the release of new virus particles from infected cells. Recently, researchers discovered that Vif (the protein encoded by the vif gene) interacts with an antiviral defense protein in host cells (APOBEC3G), causing inactivation of the antiviral effect and enhancing HIV replication. This interaction may serve as a new target for antiviral drugs.

The ends of each strand of HIV RNA contain an RNA sequence called the long terminal repeat (LTR). Regions in the LTR act as switches to control production of new viruses and can be triggered by proteins from either HIV or the host cell.

The core of HIV also includes a protein called p7, the HIV nucleocapsid protein. Three enzymes carry out later steps in the virus's life cycle: reverse transcriptase, integrase, and protease. Another HIV protein called p17, or the HIV matrix protein, lies between the viral core and the viral envelope.

REPLICATION CYCLE OF HIV

Entry of HIV into cells

Infection typically begins when an HIV particle, which contains two copies of the HIV RNA, encounters a cell with a surface molecule called cluster designation 4 (CD4). Cells carrying this molecule are known as CD4+ cells.

One or more of the virus's gp120 molecules binds tightly to CD4 molecule(s) on the cell's surface. The binding of gp120 to CD4 results in a conformational change in the gp120 molecule allowing it to bind to a second molecule on the cell surface known as a co-receptor. The envelope of the virus and the cell membrane then fuse, leading to entry of the virus into the cell. The gp41 of the envelope is critical to the fusion process. Drugs that block either the binding or the fusion process are being developed and tested in clinical trials. The Food and Drug Administration (FDA) has approved one of the so-called fusion inhibitors, T20, for use in HIV-infected people.

Simplified HIV Life Cycle

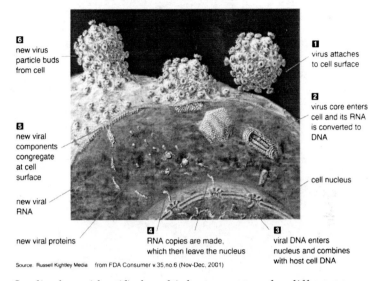

6 new virus particle buds from cell

1 virus attaches to cell surface

2 virus core enters cell and its RNA is converted to DNA

5 new viral components congregate at cell surface

cell nucleus

new viral RNA

new viral proteins

4 RNA copies are made, which then leave the nucleus

3 viral DNA enters nucleus and combines with host cell DNA

Source: Russell Kightley Media   from FDA Consumer v.35,no.6 (Nov-Dec, 2001)

Studies have identified multiple coreceptors for different types of HIV strains. These coreceptors are promising targets for new anti-HIV drugs, some of which are now being tested in preclinical and clinical studies. Agents that block the co-receptors are showing particular promise as potential microbicides that could be used in gels or creams to prevent HIV transmission. In the early stage of HIV disease, most people harbor viruses that use, in addition to CD4, a receptor called CCR5 to enter their target cells. With disease progression, the spectrum of co-receptor usage expands in approximately 50 percent of patients to include other receptors, notably a molecule called CXCR4. Virus that uses CCR5 is called R5 HIV and virus that uses CXCR4 is called X4 HIV.

Although CD4+ T cells appear to be the main targets of HIV, other immune system cells with and without CD4 molecules on their surfaces are infected as well. Among these are long-lived cells called monocytes and macrophages , which apparently can harbor large quantities of the virus without being killed, thus acting as reservoirs of HIV. CD4+ T cells also serve as important reservoirs of HIV; a small proportion of these cells harbor HIV in a

159

stable, inactive form. Normal immune processes may activate these cells, resulting in the production of new HIV virions.

Cell-to-cell spread of HIV also can occur through the CD4-mediated fusion of an infected cell with an uninfected cell.

Replication Cycle of HIV

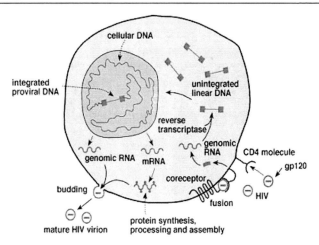

Reverse transcription

In the cytoplasm of the cell, HIV reverse transcriptase converts viral RNA into DNA, the nucleic acid form in which the cell carries its genes. Fifteen of the 26 antiviral drugs approved in the United States for treating people with HIV infection work by interfering with this stage of the viral life cycle.

Integration

The newly made HIV DNA moves to the cell's nucleus, where it is spliced into the host's DNA with the help of HIV integrase. HIV DNA that enters the DNA of the cell is called a provirus. Several drugs that target the integrase enzyme are in the early stages of development and are being investigated for their potential as antiretroviral agents.

Transcription

For a provirus to produce new viruses, RNA copies must be made that can be read by the host cell's protein-making machinery. These copies are called messenger RNA (mRNA), and production of mRNA is called transcription, a process that involves the host cell's own enzymes. Viral genes in concert with the cellular machinery control this process; the tat gene, for example, encodes a protein that accelerates transcription. Genomic RNA is also transcribed for later incorporation in the budding virion (see below).

Cytokines, proteins involved in the normal regulation of the immune response, also may regulate transcription. Molecules such as tumor necrosis factor (TNF)-alpha and interleukin (IL)-6, secreted in elevated levels by the cells of HIV-infected people, may help to activate HIV proviruses. Other infections, by organisms such as Mycobacterium tuberculosis, also may enhance transcription by inducing the secretion of cytokines.

Translation

After HIV mRNA is processed in the cell's nucleus, it is transported to the cytoplasm. HIV proteins are critical to this process; for example, a protein encoded by the rev gene allows mRNA encoding HIV structural proteins to be transferred from the nucleus to the cytoplasm. Without the rev protein, structural proteins are not made. In the cytoplasm, the virus co-opts the cell's protein-making machinery—including structures called ribosomes—to make long chains of viral proteins and enzymes, using HIV mRNA as a template. This process is called translation.

Assembly and budding

Newly made HIV core proteins, enzymes, and genomic RNA gather inside the cell and an immature viral particle forms and buds off from the cell, acquiring an envelope that includes both cellular and HIV proteins from the cell membrane. During this part of the viral life cycle, the core of the virus is immature and the virus is not yet infectious. The long chains of proteins and enzymes that make up the immature viral core are now cut into smaller pieces by a viral enzyme called protease.

This step results in infectious viral particles. Drugs called protease inhibitors interfere with this step of the viral life cycle. FDA has approved eight such drugs—saquinavir, ritonavir, indinavir, amprenavir, nelfinavir, fosamprenavir, atazanavir, and lopinavir—for marketing in the United States. Recently, an HIV inhibitor that targets a unique step in the viral life cycle, very late in the process of viral maturation, has been identified and is currently undergoing further development.

Recently, researchers have discovered that virus budding from the host cell is much more complex than previously thought. Binding between the HIV Gag protein and molecules in the cell directs the accumulation of HIV components in special intracellular sacks, called multivesicular bodies (MVB), that normally function to carry proteins out of the cell. In this way, HIV actively hitch-hikes out of the cell in the MVB by hijacking normal cell machinery and mechanisms. Discovery of this budding pathway has revealed several potential points for intervening in the viral replication cycle.

TRANSMISSION OF HIV

Among adults, HIV is spread most commonly during sexual intercourse with an infected partner. During intercourse, the virus can enter the body through the mucosal linings of the vagina, vulva, penis, or rectum or, rarely, via the mouth and possibly the upper gastrointestinal tract after oral sex. The likelihood of transmission is increased by factors that may damage these linings, especially other sexually transmitted infections that cause ulcers or inflammation.

Research suggests that immune system cells of the dendritic cell type, which live in the mucosa, may begin the infection process after sexual exposure by binding to and carrying the virus from the site of infection to the lymph nodes where other immune system cells become infected. A molecule on the surface of dendritic cells, DC-SIGN, may be critical for this transmission process.

HIV also can be transmitted by contact with infected blood, most often by the sharing of needles or syringes contaminated with minute quantities of blood containing the virus. The risk of acquiring HIV from blood transfusions is extremely small in the United States, as all blood products in this country are screened routinely for evidence of the virus.

Almost all HIV-infected children in the United States get the virus from their mothers before or during birth. In the United States, approximately 25 percent of pregnant HIV-infected women not receiving antiretroviral therapy have passed on the virus to their babies. In 1994, researchers showed that a specific regimen of the drug AZT (zidovudine) can reduce the risk of transmission of HIV from mother to baby by two-thirds. The use of combinations of antiretroviral drugs and simpler drug regimens has further reduced the rate of mother-to-child HIV transmission in the United States.

In developing countries, cheap and simple antiviral drug regimens have been proven to significantly reduce mother-to-child transmission at birth in resource-poor settings. Unfortunately, the virus also may be transmitted from an HIV-infected mother to her infant via breastfeeding. Moreover, due to the use of medicines to prevent transmission at delivery, breastfeeding may become the most common mode of HIV infection in infants. Thus, development of affordable alternatives to breastfeeding is greatly needed.

EARLY EVENTS IN HIV INFECTION

Once it enters the body, HIV infects a large number of CD4+ cells and replicates rapidly. During this acute or primary phase of infection, the blood contains many viral particles that spread throughout the body, seeding various organs, particularly the lymphoid organs.

Two to 4 weeks after exposure to the virus, up to 70 percent of HIV-infected people suffer flu-like symptoms related to the acute infection. Their immune system fights back with killer T cells (CD8+ T cells) and B-cell-produced antibodies , which dramatically reduce HIV levels. A person's CD4+ T cell count may rebound somewhat and even approach its original level. A person may then remain free of HIV-related symptoms for years despite continuous replication of HIV in the lymphoid organs that had been seeded during the acute phase of infection.

One reason that HIV is unique is the fact that despite the body's aggressive immune responses, which are sufficient to clear most viral infections, some HIV invariably escapes. This is due in large part to the high rate of mutations that occur during the process of HIV replication. Even when the virus does not avoid the immune system by mutating, the body's best soldiers in the fight against HIV—certain subsets of killer T cells that recognize HIV—may be depleted or become dysfunctional.

In addition, early in the course of HIV infection, people may lose HIV-specific CD4+ T cell responses that normally slow the replication of viruses. Such responses include the secretion of interferons and other antiviral factors, and the orchestration of CD8+ T cells.

Finally, the virus may hide within the chromosomes of an infected cell and be shielded from surveillance by the immune system. Such cells can be considered as a latent reservoir of the virus. Because the antiviral agents currently in our therapeutic arsenal attack actively replicating virus, they are not effective against hidden, inactive viral DNA (so-called provirus). New strategies to purge this latent reservoir of HIV have become one of the major goals for current research efforts.

COURSE OF HIV INFECTION

Among people enrolled in large epidemiologic studies in Western countries, the median time from infection with HIV to the development of AIDS-related symptoms has been approximately 10 to 12 years in the absence of antiretroviral therapy. Researchers, however, have observed a wide variation in disease progression. Approximately 10 percent of HIV-infected people in these studies have progressed to AIDS within the first 2 to 3 years following infection, while up to 5 percent of individuals in the studies have stable CD4+ T cell counts and no symptoms even after 12 or more years.

Factors such as age or genetic differences among individuals, the level of virulence of an individual strain of virus, and co-infection with other microbes may influence the rate and severity of disease progression. Drugs that fight the infections associated with AIDS have improved and prolonged the lives of HIV-infected people by preventing or treating conditions such as Pneumocystis carinii pneumonia, cytomegalovirus disease, and diseases caused by a number of fungi.

HIV co-receptors and disease progression

Recent research has shown that most infecting strains of HIV use a co-receptor molecule called CCR5, in addition to the CD4 molecule, to enter certain of its target cells. HIV-infected people with a specific mutation in one of their two copies of the gene for this receptor may have a slower disease course than people with two normal copies of the gene. Rare individuals with two mutant copies of the CCR5 gene appear, in most cases, to be completely protected from HIV infection. Mutations in the gene for other HIV co-receptors also may influence the rate of disease progression.

Viral burden and disease progression

Numerous studies show that people with high levels of HIV in their bloodstream are more likely to develop new AIDS-related symptoms or die than those with lower levels of virus. For instance, in the Multicenter AIDS Cohort Study (MACS), investigators showed that the level of HIV in an untreated person's plasma 6 months to a year after infection—the so-called viral "set point"—is highly predictive of the rate of disease progression; that is, patients with high levels of virus are much more likely to get sicker faster than those with low levels of virus. The MACS and other studies have provided the rationale for providing aggressive antiretroviral therapy to HIV-infected people, as well as for routinely using newly available blood tests to measure viral load when initiating, monitoring, and modifying anti-HIV therapy.

Potent combinations of three or more anti-HIV drugs known as highly active antiretroviral therapy, or HAART, can reduce a person's "viral burden" (amount of virus in the circulating blood) to very low levels and in many cases delay the progression of HIV disease for prolonged periods. Before the introduction of HAART therapy, 85 percent of patients survived an average of 3 years following AIDS diagnosis. Today, 95 percent of patients who start therapy before they get AIDS survive on average 3 years following their first AIDS diagnosis. For those who start HAART after their

165

first AIDS event, survival is still very high at 85 percent, averaging 3 years after AIDS diagnosis.

Antiretroviral regimens, however, have yet to completely and permanently suppress the virus in HIV-infected people. Recent studies have shown that, in addition to the latent HIV reservoir discussed above, HIV persists in a replication-competent form in resting CD4+ T cells even in people receiving aggressive antiretroviral therapy who have no readily detectable HIV in their blood. Investigators around the world are working to develop the next generation of anti-HIV drugs that can stop HIV, even in these biological scenarios.

A treatment goal, along with reduction of viral burden, is the reconstitution of the person's immune system, which may have become sufficiently damaged that it cannot replenish itself. Various strategies for assisting the immune system in this regard are being tested in clinical trials in tandem with HAART, such as the Evaluation of Subcutaneous Proleukin in a Randomized International Trial (ESPRIT) trial exploring the effects of the T cell growth factor, IL-2.

HIV IS ACTIVE IN THE LYMPH NODES

Although HIV-infected people often show an extended period of clinical latency with little evidence of disease, the virus is never truly completely latent although individual cells may be latently infected. Researchers have shown that even early in disease, HIV actively replicates within the lymph nodes and related organs, where large amounts of virus become trapped in networks of specialized cells with long, tentacle-like extensions. These cells are called follicular dendritic cells (FDCs). FDCs are located in hot spots of immune activity in lymphoid tissue called germinal centers. They act like flypaper, trapping invading pathogens (including HIV) and holding them until B cells come along to start an immune response.

Over a period of years, even when little virus is readily detectable in the blood, significant amounts of virus accumulate in the lymphoid tissue, both within infected cells and bound to FDCs. In and around the germinal centers, numerous CD4+ T cells are probably activated by the increased production of cytokines such as TNF-alpha and IL-6 by immune system cells within the lymphoid tissue. Activation allows uninfected cells to be more easily infected and increases replication of HIV in already infected cells.

While greater quantities of certain cytokines such as TNF-alpha and IL-6 are secreted during HIV infection, other cytokines with key roles in the regulation of normal immune function may be secreted in decreased amounts. For example, CD4+ T cells may lose their capacity to produce IL-2, a cytokine that enhances the growth of other T cells and helps to stimulate other cells' response to invaders. Infected cells also have low levels of receptors for IL-2, which may reduce their ability to respond to signals from other cells.

Breakdown of lymph node architecture

Ultimately, with chronic cell activation and secretion of inflammatory cytokines, the fine and complex inner structure of the lymph node breaks down and is replaced by scar tissue. Without this structure, cells in the lymph node cannot communicate and the immune system cannot function properly. Investigators also have reported recently that this scarring reduces the ability of the immune system to replenish itself following antiretroviral therapy that reduces the viral burden.

ROLE OF CD8+ T CELLS

CD8+ T cells are critically important in the immune response to HIV. These cells attack and kill infected cells that are producing virus. Thus, vaccine efforts are directed toward eliciting or enhancing these killer T cells, as well as eliciting antibodies that will neutralize the infectivity of HIV.

CD8+ T cells also appear to secrete soluble factors that suppress HIV replication. Several molecules, including RANTES, MIP-1alpha, MIP-1beta, and MDC appear to block HIV replication by occupying the coreceptors necessary for many strains of HIV to enter their target cells. There may be other immune system molecules—including the so-called CD8 antiviral factor (CAF), the defensins (type of antimicrobials), and others yet undiscovered—that can suppress HIV replication to some degree.

RAPID REPLICATION AND MUTATION OF HIV

HIV replicates rapidly; several billion new virus particles may be produced every day. In addition, the HIV reverse transcriptase enzyme makes many mistakes while making DNA copies from HIV RNA. As a consequence, many variants or strains of HIV develop in a person, some of which may escape destruction by antibodies or killer T cells. Additionally, different strains of HIV can recombine to produce a wide range of variants.

During the course of HIV disease, viral strains emerge in an infected person that differ widely in their ability to infect and kill different cell types, as well as in their rate of replication. Scientists are investigating why strains of HIV from people with advanced disease appear to be more virulent and infect more cell types than strains obtained earlier from the same person. Part of the explanation may be the expanded ability of the virus to use other co-receptors, such as CXCR4.

THEORIES OF IMMUNE SYSTEM CELL LOSS IN HIV INFECTION

Researchers around the world are studying how HIV destroys or disables CD4+ T cells, and many think that a number of mechanisms may occur simultaneously in an HIV-infected person. Data suggest that billions of CD4+ T cells may be destroyed every day, eventually overwhelming the immune system's capacity to regenerate.

Direct cell killing

Infected CD4+ T cells may be killed directly when large amounts of virus are produced and bud out from the cell surface, disrupting the cell membrane, or when viral proteins and nucleic acids collect inside the cell, interfering with cellular machinery.

Apoptosis

Infected CD4+ T cells may be killed when the regulation of cell function is distorted by HIV proteins, probably leading to cell suicide by a process known as programmed cell death or apoptosis. Recent reports indicate that apoptosis occurs to a greater extent in HIV-infected people, both in their bloodstream and lymph nodes.

Apoptosis is closely associated with the aberrant cellular activation seen in HIV disease.

Uninfected cells also may undergo apoptosis. Investigators have shown in cell cultures that the HIV envelope alone or bound to antibodies sends an inappropriate signal to CD4+ T cells causing them to undergo apoptosis, even if not infected by HIV.

Innocent bystanders

Uninfected cells may die in an innocent bystander scenario: HIV particles may bind to the cell surface, giving them the appearance of an infected cell and marking them for destruction by killer T cells after antibody attaches to the viral particle on the cell. This process is called antibody-dependent cellular cytotoxicity.

Killer T cells also may mistakenly destroy uninfected cells that have consumed HIV particles and that display HIV fragments on their surfaces. Alternatively, because HIV envelope proteins bear some resemblance to certain molecules that may appear on CD4+ T cells, the body's immune responses may mistakenly damage such cells as well.

Anergy

Researchers have shown in cell cultures that CD4+ T cells can be turned off by activation signals from HIV that leaves them unable to respond to further immune stimulation. This inactivated state is known as anergy.

Damage to precursor cells

Studies suggest that HIV also destroys precursor cells that mature to have special immune functions, as well as the microenvironment of the bone marrow and the thymus needed for developing such cells. These organs probably lose the ability to regenerate, further compounding the suppression of the immune system.

CENTRAL NERVOUS SYSTEM DAMAGE

Although monocytes and macrophages can be infected by HIV, they appear to be relatively resistant to being killed by the virus. These cells, however, travel throughout the body and carry HIV to various organs, including the brain, which may serve as a hiding place or "reservoir" for the virus that may be relatively resistant to most anti-HIV drugs.

Neurologic manifestations of HIV disease are seen in up to 50 percent of HIV-infected people, to varying degrees of severity. People infected with HIV often experience

Cognitive symptoms, including impaired short-term memory, reduced concentration, and mental slowing

Motor symptoms such as fine motor clumsiness or slowness, tremor, and leg weakness

Behavioral symptoms including apathy, social withdrawal, irritability, depression, and personality change

More serious neurologic manifestations in HIV disease typically occur in patients with high viral loads, generally when a person has advanced HIV disease or AIDS.

Neurologic manifestations of HIV disease are the subject of many research projects. Current evidence suggests that although nerve cells do not become infected with HIV, supportive cells within the brain, such as astrocytes and microglia (as well as monocyte/macrophages that have migrated to the brain) can be infected with the virus. Researchers postulate that infection of these cells can cause a disruption of normal neurologic functions by altering cytokine levels, by delivering aberrant signals, and by causing the release of toxic products in the brain. The use of anti-HIV drugs frequently reduces the severity of neurologic symptoms, but in many cases does not, for reasons that are unclear. The impact of long-term therapy and long-term HIV disease on neurologic function is also unknown and under intensive study.

ROLE OF IMMUNE ACTIVATION IN HIV DISEASE

During a normal immune response, many parts of the immune system are mobilized to fight an invader. CD4+ T cells, for instance, may quickly multiply and increase their cytokine secretion, thereby signaling other cells to perform their special functions. Scavenger cells called macrophages may double in size and develop numerous organelles , including lysosomes that contain digestive enzymes used to process ingested pathogens. Once the immune system clears the foreign antigen, it returns to a relative state of quiescence.

Paradoxically, although it ultimately causes immune deficiency, HIV disease for most of its course is characterized by immune system hyperactivation, which has negative consequences. As noted above, HIV replication and spread are much more efficient in activated CD4+ cells. Chronic immune system activation during HIV disease also may result in a massive stimulation of B cells, impairing the ability of these cells to make antibodies against other pathogens.

Chronic immune activation also can result in apoptosis, and an increased production of cytokines that not only may increase HIV replication but also have other deleterious effects. Increased levels of TNF-alpha, for example, may be at least partly responsible for the severe weight loss or wasting syndrome seen in many HIV-infected people.

The persistence of HIV and HIV replication plays an important role in the chronic state of immune activation seen in HIV-infected people. In addition, researchers have shown that infections with other organisms activate immune system cells and increase production of the virus in HIV-infected people. Chronic immune activation due to persistent infections, or the cumulative effects of multiple episodes of immune activation and bursts of virus production, likely contribute to the progression of HIV disease.

NEW CLINICAL SIGNS OF HIV IN THE ERA OF HAART THERAPY

The clinical spectrum of disease among people with HIV has changed dramatically in the era of HAART. NIAID and its grantees are actively studying the new clinical syndrome of disease among persons on long term-therapy. Research is concentrating on the impact of HIV over the long term, the toxicity of the medicines used to control HIV, and the effects of aging on HIV disease progression. People with HIV have a variety of conditions including diabetes, heart disease, neurocognitive decline, and cancers that may, or may not, be directly due to HIV or its treatment.

171

Long-term studies of people with HIV in the United States and abroad are underway.

NIAID RESEARCH ON THE PATHOGENESIS OF AIDS

NIAID-supported scientists conduct research on HIV pathogenesis in laboratories on the campus of the National Institutes of Health (NIH) in Bethesda, Maryland; at the Institute's Rocky Mountain Laboratories in Hamilton, Montana; and at universities and medical centers in the United States and abroad.

An NIAID-supported resource, the NIH AIDS Research and Reference Reagent Program , in collaboration with the World Health Organization, provides critically needed AIDS-related research materials free to qualified researchers around the world.

The NIH Centers for AIDS Research , supported by NIAID in collaboration with six other NIH Institutes, fosters and facilitates development of infrastructure and interdisciplinary collaboration of HIV researchers at major medical and research centers across the United States.

In addition, the Institute convenes groups of investigators and advisory committees to exchange scientific information, clarify research priorities, and bring research needs and opportunities to the attention of the scientific community.

GLOSSARY

antibodies - infection-fighting protein molecules in blood or secretory fluids that tag, neutralize, and help destroy pathogenic microorganisms such as viruses.

apoptosis - cellular suicide, also known as programmed cell death. HIV may induce apoptosis in both infected and uninfected immune system cells.

B cells - white blood cells of the immune system that produce infection-fighting proteins called antibodies.

CD4+ T cells - white blood cells that orchestrate the immune response, signaling other cells in the immune system to perform their special functions. Also known as T helper cells, these cells are killed or disabled during HIV infection.

CD8+ T cells - white blood cells that kill cells infected with HIV or other viruses, or transformed by cancer. These cells also secrete soluble molecules that may suppress HIV without killing infected cells directly.

cytokines - proteins used for communication by cells of the immune system. Central to the normal regulation of the immune response.

cytoplasm - the living matter within a cell.

dendritic cells - immune system cells with long, tentacle-like branches. Some of these are specialized cells at the mucosa that may bind to HIV following sexual exposure and carry the virus from the site of infection to the lymph nodes. See also follicular dendritic cells.

enzyme - a protein that accelerates a specific chemical reaction without altering itself.

follicular dendritic cells (FDCs) - cells found in the germinal centers (B cell areas) of lymphoid organs. FDCs have thread-like tentacles that form a web-like network to trap invaders and present them to B cells, which then make antibodies to attack the invaders.

germinal centers - structures within lymphoid tissues that contain FDCs and B cells, and in which immune responses are initiated.

gp41 - glycoprotein 41, a protein embedded in the outer envelope of HIV. Plays a key role in HIV's infection of CD4+ T cells by facilitating the fusion of the viral and cell membranes.

gp120 - glycoprotein 120, a protein that protrudes from the surface of HIV and binds to CD4+ T cells.

gp160 - glycoprotein 160, an HIV precursor protein that is cleaved by the HIV protease enzyme into gp41 and gp120.

immune deficiency - the inability of the immune system to work properly, resulting in susceptibility to disease.

immunosuppression - immune system response to foreign invaders such as HIV is reduced

integrase - an HIV enzyme used by the virus to integrate its genetic material into the host cell's DNA.

Kaposi's sarcoma - a type of cancer characterized by abnormal growths of blood vessels that develop into purplish or brown lesions.

killer T cells - see CD8+ T cells.

lentivirus - "slow" virus characterized by a long interval between infection and the onset of symptoms. HIV is a lentivirus as is the simian immunodeficiency virus (SIV), which infects non-human primates.

LTR - long terminal repeat, the RNA sequences repeated at both ends of HIV's genetic material. These regulatory switches may help control viral transcription.

lymphoid organs - include tonsils, adenoids, lymph nodes, spleen, and other tissues. Act as the body's filtering system, trapping invaders and presenting them to squadrons of immune cells that congregate there.

macrophage - a large immune system cell that devours invading pathogens and other intruders. Stimulates other immune system cells by presenting them with small pieces of the invaders.

microbes - microscopic living organisms, including viruses, bacteria, fungi, and protozoa.

monocyte - a circulating white blood cell that develops into a macrophage when it enters tissues.

opportunistic infection - an illness caused by an organism that usually does not cause disease in a person with a normal immune system. People with advanced HIV infection suffer opportunistic infections of the lungs, brain, eyes, and other organs.

organelles - small structures inside a cell, generally bounded by membranes.

pathogenesis - the production or development of a disease. May be influenced by many factors, including the infecting microbe and the host's immune response.

pathogens - disease-causing organisms.

protease - an HIV enzyme used to cut large HIV proteins into smaller ones needed for the assembly of an infectious virus particle.

provirus - DNA of a virus, such as HIV, that has been integrated into the genes of a host cell.

replicate: process by which a virus makes copies of itself.

retrovirus - HIV and other viruses that carry their genetic material in the form of RNA and that have the enzyme reverse transcriptase.

reverse transcriptase - the enzyme produced by HIV and other retroviruses that allows them to synthesize DNA from their RNA.

Human Immunodeficiency Virus Type 2

In 1984, 3 years after the first reports of a disease that was to become known as AIDS, researchers discovered the primary causative viral agent, the human immunodeficiency virus type 1 (HIV-1). In 1986, a second type of HIV, called HIV-2, was isolated from AIDS patients in West Africa, where it may have been present decades earlier. Studies of the natural history of HIV-2 are limited, but to date comparisons with HIV-1 show some similarities while suggesting differences. Both HIV-1 and HIV-2 have the same modes of transmission and are associated with similar opportunistic infections and AIDS. In persons infected with HIV-2, immunodeficiency seems to develop more slowly and to be milder. Compared with persons infected with HIV-1, those with HIV-2 are less infectious early in the course of infection. As the disease advances, HIV-2 infectiousness seems to increase; however, compared with HIV-1, the duration of this increased infectiousness is shorter. HIV-1 and HIV-2 also differ in geographic patterns of infection; the United States has few reported cases.

175

Which countries have a high prevalence* of HIV-2 infection?

HIV-2 infections are predominantly found in Africa. West African nations with a prevalence of HIV-2 of more than 1% in the general population are Cape Verde, Côte d'Ivoire (Ivory Coast), Gambia, Guinea-Bissau, Mali, Mauritania, Nigeria, and Sierra Leone. Other West African countries reporting HIV-2 are Benin, Burkina Faso, Ghana, Guinea, Liberia, Niger, São Tomé, Senegal, and Togo. Angola and Mozambique are other African nations where the prevalence of HIV-2 is more than 1%.

What is known about HIV-2 in the United States?

The first case of HIV-2 infection in the United States was diagnosed in 1987. Since then, the Centers for Disease Control and Prevention (CDC) has worked with state and local health departments to collect demographic, clinical, and laboratory data on persons with HIV-2 infection.

Of the 79 infected persons, 66 are black and 51 are male. Fifty-two were born in West Africa, 1 in Kenya, 7 in the United States, 2 in India, and 2 in Europe. The region of origin was not known for 15 of the persons, although 4 of them had a malaria-antibody profile consistent with residence in West Africa. AIDS-defining conditions have developed in 17, and 8 have died.

These case counts represent minimal estimates because completeness of reporting has not been assessed. Although AIDS is reported uniformly nationwide, the reporting of HIV infection, including HIV-2 infection, differs from state to state according to state policy.

Who should be tested for HIV-2?

Because epidemiologic data indicate that the prevalence of HIV-2 in the United States is very low, CDC does not recommend routine HIV-2 testing at U.S. HIV counseling and test sites or in settings other than blood centers. However, when HIV testing is to be performed, tests for antibodies to both HIV-1 and HIV-2 should be obtained if demographic or behavioral information suggests that HIV-2 infection might be present.

Persons at risk for HIV-2 infection include

176

- Sex partners of a person from a country where HIV-2 is endemic (refer to countries listed earlier)
- Sex partners of a person known to be infected with HIV-2
- People who received a blood transfusion or a non-sterile injection in a country where HIV-2 is endemic
- People who shared needles with a person from a country where HIV-2 is endemic or with a person known to be infected with HIV-2
- Children of women who have risk factors for HIV-2 infection or are known to be infected with HIV-2

HIV-2 testing also is indicated for
- People with an illness that suggests HIV infection (such as an HIV-associated opportunistic infection) but whose HIV-1 test result is not positive
- People for whom HIV-1 Western blot exhibits the unusual indeterminate test band pattern of gag (p55, p24, or p17) plus pol (p66, p51, or p32) in the absence of env (gp160, gp120, or gp41)

Among all HIV-infected people, the prevalence of HIV-2 is very low compared with HIV-1. However, the potential risk for HIV-2 infection in some populations (such as those listed) may justify routine HIV-2 testing for all people for whom HIV-1 testing is warranted. The decision to implement routine HIV-2 testing requires consideration of the number of HIV-2-infected persons whose infection would remain undiagnosed without routine HIV-2 testing compared with the problems and costs associated with the implementation of HIV-2 testing.

The development of antibodies is similar in HIV-1 and HIV-2. Antibodies generally become detectable within 3 months of infection. Testing for HIV-2 antibodies is available through private physicians or state and local health departments.

Are blood donors tested for HIV-2?

Since 1992, all U.S. blood donations have been tested with a combination HIV-1/HIV-2 enzyme immunoassay test kit that is sensitive to antibodies to both viruses. This testing has demonstrated that HIV-2 infection in blood donors is extremely rare. All donations detected with either HIV-1 or HIV-2 are excluded from any clinical use, and donors are deferred from further donations.

Is the clinical treatment of HIV-2 different from that of HIV-1?

Little is known about the best approach to the clinical treatment and care of patients infected with HIV-2. Given the slower development of immunodeficiency and the limited clinical experience with HIV-2, it is unclear whether antiretroviral therapy significantly slows progression. Not all of the drugs used to treat HIV-1 infection are as effective against HIV-2. In vitro (laboratory) studies suggest that nucleoside analogs are active against HIV-2, though not as active as against HIV-1. Protease inhibitors should be active against HIV-2. However, non-nucleoside reverse transcriptase inhibitors (NNRTIs) are not active against HIV-2. Whether any potential benefits would outweigh the possible adverse effects of treatment is unknown.

Monitoring the treatment response of patients infected with HIV-2 is more difficult than monitoring people infected with HIV-1. No FDA-licensed HIV-2 viral load assay is available yet. Viral load assays used for HIV-1 are not reliable for monitoring HIV-2. Response to treatment for HIV-2 infection may be monitored by following CD4+ T-cell counts and other indicators of immune system deterioration, such as weight loss, oral candidiasis, unexplained fever, and the appearance of a new AIDS-defining illness. More research and clinical experience is needed to determine the most effective treatment for HIV-2.

The optimal timing for antiretroviral therapy (i.e., soon after infection, when symptoms appear, or when CD4+ T cell counts fall below a certain level) remains under review by clinical experts. Guidelines for the Use of Antiretroviral Agents in HIV-Infected Adults and Adolescents, by the Department of Health and Human Services Panel on Clinical Practices for Treatment of HIV Infection, may be helpful to the clinician who is caring for a patient infected with HIV-2; however, the recommendations on viral load monitoring and the use of NNRTIs would not apply to patients with HIV-2 infection. Copies of the guidelines are available from the CDC National Prevention Information Network (1 800 458-5231) and from its Web site (www.cdcnpin.org). The guidelines also are available from the HIV/AIDS Treatment Information Service (1 800 448-0440; Fax 301 519-6616; TTY 1 800 243-7012) and on the ATIS Web site (www.hivatis.org).

What is known about HIV-2 infection in children?

HIV-2 infection in children is rare. Compared with HIV-1, HIV-2 seems to be less transmissible from an infected mother to her child. However, cases of transmission from an infected woman to her fetus or newborn have been reported among women who had primary HIV-2 infection during their pregnancy. Zidovudine therapy has been demonstrated to reduce the risk for perinatal HIV-1 transmission and also might prove effective for reducing perinatal HIV-2 transmission. Zidovudine therapy should be considered for HIV-2-infected expectant mothers and their newborns, especially for women who become infected during pregnancy.

How should physicians and patients decide whether to start treatment for HIV-2?

Physicians caring for patients with HIV-2 infection should decide whether to initiate antiretroviral therapy after discussing with their patients what is known, what is not known, and the possible adverse effects of treatment.

What can be done to control the spread of HIV-2?

Continued surveillance is needed to monitor HIV-2 in the U.S. population because the possibility for further spread of HIV-2 exists, especially among injecting drug users and people with multiple sex partners. Programs aimed at preventing the transmission of HIV-1 also can help to prevent and control the spread of HIV-2.

Frequently Asked Questions on Human Immunodeficiency Virus (HIV) and Acquired Immunodeficiency Syndrome (AIDS)

What is HIV?

HIV (human immunodeficiency virus) is the virus that causes AIDS. This virus may be passed from one person to another when infected blood, semen, or vaginal secretions come in contact with an uninfected person's broken skin or mucous membranes. (A mucous membrane is wet, thin tissue found in certain openings to the human body. These can include the mouth, eyes, nose, vagina, rectum, and opening of the penis.)

In addition, infected pregnant women can pass HIV to their baby during pregnancy or delivery, as well as through breast-feeding. People with HIV have what is called HIV infection. Some of these people will develop AIDS as a result of their HIV infection.

What is AIDS?

AIDS stands for Acquired Immunodeficiency Syndrome.

Acquired – means that the disease is not hereditary but develops after birth from contact with a disease causing agent (in this case, HIV).

Immunodeficiency – means that the disease is characterized by a weakening of the immune system.

Syndrome – refers to a group of symptoms that collectively indicate or characterize a disease. In the case of AIDS this can include the development of certain infections and/or cancers, as well as a decrease in the number of certain cells in a person's immune system.

A diagnosis of AIDS is made by a physician using specific clinical or laboratory standards.

Where did HIV come from?

The earliest known case of HIV-1 in a human was from a blood sample collected in 1959 from a man in Kinshasa, Democratic Republic of Congo. (How he became infected is not known.) Genetic analysis of this blood sample suggested that HIV-1 may have stemmed from a single virus in the late 1940s or early 1950s.

We know that the virus has existed in the United States since at least the mid- to late 1970s. From 1979-1981 rare types of pneumonia, cancer, and other illnesses were being reported by doctors in Los Angeles and New York among a number of male patients who had sex with other men. These were conditions not usually found in people with healthy immune systems.

In 1982 public health officials began to use the term "acquired immunodeficiency syndrome," or AIDS, to describe the occurrences of opportunistic infections, Kaposi's sarcoma (a kind of cancer), and Pneumocystis carinii pneumonia in previously healthy people. Formal tracking (surveillance) of AIDS cases began that year in the United States.

In 1983, scientists discovered the virus that causes AIDS. The virus was at first named HTLV-III/LAV (human T-cell lymphotropic virus-type III/lymphadenopathy- associated virus) by an international scientific committee. This name was later changed to HIV (human immunodeficiency virus).

For many years scientists theorized as to the origins of HIV and how it appeared in the human population, most believing that HIV originated in other primates. Then in 1999, an international team of researchers reported that they had discovered the origins of HIV-1, the predominant strain of HIV in the developed world. A subspecies of chimpanzees native to west equatorial Africa had been identified as the original source of the virus. The researchers believe that HIV-1 was introduced into the human population when hunters became exposed to infected blood.

What causes AIDS?

AIDS is caused by infection with a virus called human immunodeficiency virus (HIV). This virus is passed from one person to another through blood-to-blood and sexual contact. In addition, infected pregnant women can pass HIV to their babies during pregnancy or delivery, as well as through breast feeding. People with HIV have what is called HIV infection. Some of these people will develop AIDS as a result of their HIV infection.

How does HIV cause AIDS?

HIV destroys a certain kind of blood cell (CD4+ T cells) which is crucial to the normal function of the human immune system. In fact, loss of these cells in people with HIV is an extremely powerful predictor of the development of AIDS. Studies of thousands of people have revealed that most people infected with HIV carry the virus for years before enough damage is done to the immune system for AIDS to develop. However, sensitive tests have shown a strong connection between the amount of HIV in the blood and the decline in CD4+ T cells and the development of AIDS. Reducing the amount of virus in the body with anti-retroviral therapies can dramatically slow the destruction of a person's immune system.

How long does it take for HIV to cause AIDS?

Prior to 1996, scientists estimated that about half the people with HIV would develop AIDS within 10 years after becoming infected. This time varied greatly from person to person and depended on many factors, including a person's health status and their health-related behaviors.

Since 1996, the introduction of powerful anti-retroviral therapies has dramatically changed the progression time between HIV infection and the development of AIDS. There are also other medical treatments that can prevent or cure some of the illnesses associated with AIDS, though the treatments do not cure AIDS itself. Because of these advances in drug therapies and other medical treatments, estimates of how many people will develop AIDS and how soon are being recalculated, revised, or are currently under study.

As with other diseases, early detection of infection allows for more options for treatment and preventative health care.

Why do some people make statements that HIV does not cause AIDS?

The epidemic of HIV and AIDS has attracted much attention both within and outside the medical and scientific communities. Much of this attention comes from the many social issues related to this disease such as sexuality, drug use, and poverty. Although the scientific evidence is overwhelming and compelling that HIV is the cause of AIDS, the disease process is still not completely understood. This incomplete understanding has led some persons to make statements that AIDS is not caused by an infectious agent or is caused by a virus that is not HIV. This is not only misleading, but may have dangerous consequences. Before the discovery of HIV, evidence from epidemiologic studies involving tracing of patients' sex partners and cases occurring in persons receiving transfusions of blood or blood clotting products had clearly indicated that the underlying cause of the condition was an infectious agent. Infection with HIV has been the sole common factor shared by AIDS cases throughout the world among men who have sex with men, transfusion recipients, persons with hemophilia, sex partners of infected persons, children born to infected women, and occupationally exposed health care workers.

The conclusion after more than 20 years of scientific research is that people, if exposed to HIV through sexual contact or injecting drug use for example, may become infected with HIV. If they become infected, most will eventually develop AIDS.

How well does HIV survive outside the body?

Scientists and medical authorities agree that HIV does not survive well outside the body, making the possibility of environmental transmission remote. HIV is found in varying concentrations or amounts in blood, semen, vaginal fluid, breast milk, saliva, and tears. To obtain data on the survival of HIV, laboratory studies have required the use of artificially high concentrations of laboratory-grown virus. Although these unnatural concentrations of HIV can be kept alive for days or even weeks under precisely controlled and limited laboratory conditions, CDC studies have shown that drying of even these high concentrations of HIV reduces the amount of infectious virus by 90 to 99 percent within several hours. Since the HIV concentrations used in laboratory studies are much higher than those actually found in blood or other specimens, drying of HIV-infected human blood or other body fluids reduces the theoretical risk of environmental transmission to that which has been observed - essentially zero. Incorrect interpretations of conclusions drawn from laboratory studies have in some instances caused unnecessary alarm.

Results from laboratory studies should not be used to assess specific personal risk of infection because

- the amount of virus studied is not found in human specimens or elsewhere in nature, and
- no one has been identified as infected with HIV due to contact with an environmental surface. Additionally, HIV is unable to reproduce outside its living host (unlike many bacteria or fungi, which may do so under suitable conditions), except under laboratory conditions; therefore, it does not spread or maintain infectiousness outside its host.

How can I tell if I'm infected with HIV? What are the symptoms?

The only way to know if you are infected is to be tested for HIV infection. You cannot rely on symptoms to know whether or not you are infected. Many people who are infected with HIV do not have any symptoms at all for many years.

The following may be warning signs of HIV infection:

- rapid weight loss
- dry cough
- recurring fever or profuse night sweats
- profound and unexplained fatigue
- swollen lymph glands in the armpits, groin, or neck
- diarrhea that lasts for more than a week

184

- white spots or unusual blemishes on the tongue, in the mouth, or in the throat
- pneumonia
- red, brown, pink, or purplish blotches on or under the skin or inside the mouth, nose, or eyelids
- memory loss, depression, and other neurological disorders

However, no one should assume they are infected if they have any of these symptoms. Each of these symptoms can be related to other illnesses. Again, the only way to determine whether you are infected is to be tested for HIV infection. For information on where to find an HIV testing site, visit the National HIV Testing Resources Web site at http://www.hivtest.org or call CDC-INFO 24 Hours/Day at1-800-CDC-INFO (232-4636), 1-888-232-6348 (TTY), in English, en Español.

You also cannot rely on symptoms to establish that a person has AIDS. The symptoms of AIDS are similar to the symptoms of many other illnesses. AIDS is a medical diagnosis made by a doctor based on specific criteria established by the CDC. For more information refer to the Morbidity and Mortality Weekly Report " 1993 Revised Classification System for HIV Infection and Expanded Surveillance Case Definition for AIDS Among Adolescents and Adults

What are the different HIV screening tests available in the U.S.?

In most cases the EIA (enzyme immunoassay), performed on blood drawn from a vein, is the standard screening test used to detect the presence of antibodies to HIV. A reactive EIA must be used with a follow-up confirmatory test such as the Western blot to make a positive diagnosis. There are EIA tests that use other body fluids to screen for antibodies to HIV. These include:

- Oral Fluid Tests – use oral fluid (not saliva) that is collected from the mouth using a special collection device. This is an EIA antibody test similar to the standard blood EIA test and requires a follow-up confirmatory Western Blot using the same oral fluid sample.

- Urine Tests – use urine instead of blood. The sensitivity and specificity (accuracy) are somewhat less than that of the blood and oral fluid tests. This is also an EIA antibody test similar to blood EIA tests and requires a follow-up confirmatory Western Blot using the same urine sample.

Rapid Tests:

A rapid test is a screening test that produces very quick results, in approximately 20-60 minutes. Rapid tests use blood or oral fluid to look for the presence of antibodies to HIV. As is true for all screening tests, a reactive rapid HIV test result must be confirmed with a follow-up confirmatory test before a final diagnosis of infection can be made. These tests have similar accuracy rates as traditional EIA screening tests. Please visit the rapid HIV testing section of the Divisions of HIV/AIDS Prevention Web site for details.

Home Testing Kits:

Consumer-controlled test kits (popularly known as "home testing kits") were first licensed in 1997. Although home HIV tests are sometimes advertised through the Internet, currently only the Home Access HIV-1 Test System is approved by the Food and Drug Administration. (The accuracy of other home test kits cannot be verified). The Home Access HIV-1 Test System can be found at most local drug stores. It is not a true home test, but a home collection kit. The testing procedure involves pricking a finger with a special device, placing drops of blood on a specially treated card, and then mailing the card in to be tested at a licensed laboratory. Customers are given an identification number to use when phoning in for the results. Callers may speak to a counselor before taking the test, while waiting for the test result, and when the results are given. All individuals receiving a positive test result are provided referrals for a follow-up confirmatory test, as well as information and resources on treatment and support services.

186

There are other tests that are used in screening the blood supply and for rare cases when standard tests are unable to detect antibodies to HIV.

How long after a possible exposure should I wait to get tested for HIV?

It can take some time for the immune system to produce enough antibodies for the antibody test to detect and this time period can vary from person to person. This time period is commonly referred to as the "window period". Most people will develop detectable antibodies within 2 to 8 weeks (the average is 25 days). Even so, there is a chance that some individuals will take longer to develop detectable antibodies. Therefore, if the initial negative HIV test was conducted within the first 3 months after possible exposure, repeat testing should be considered >3 months after the exposure occurred to account for the possibility of a false-negative result. Ninety seven percent will develop antibodies in the first 3 months following the time of their infection. In very rare cases, it can take up to 6 months to develop antibodies to HIV.

Where can I get tested for HIV infection?

Many places provide testing for HIV infection. Common testing locations include local health departments, clinics, offices of private doctors, hospitals, and other sites set up specifically to provide HIV testing

Between the time of a possible exposure and the receipt of test results, individuals should consider abstaining from sexual contact with others or use condoms and/or dental dams during all sexual encounters.

It is important to seek testing at a place that also provides counseling about HIV prevention and AIDS. Counselors can answer any questions you might have about risky behaviors and ways you can protect yourself and others in the future. In addition, they can help you understand the meaning of the test results and describe what HIV/AIDS-related resources are available in the local area.

187

If I test HIV negative, does that mean that my partner is HIV negative also?

No. Your HIV test result reveals only your HIV status. Your negative test result does not indicate whether or not your partner has HIV. HIV is not necessarily transmitted every time there is an exposure. Therefore, your taking an HIV test should not be seen as a method to find out if your partner is infected.

Ask your partner about his or her HIV status; what risk behaviors they have engaged in both currently and in the past; and encourage your partner to get tested for HIV.

It is important to take steps to reduce your risk of getting HIV. Not having (abstaining from) sex is the most effective way to avoid HIV. If you choose to be sexually active, mutually monogamous sex with an uninfected partner is also effective. If you choose to have sex with a partner where either you or your partner's HIV status is uncertain, use a latex condom to help protect both you and your partner from HIV and other STDs. Studies have shown that latex condoms are very effective, though not 100%, in preventing HIV transmission when used correctly and consistently. If either partner is allergic to latex, plastic (polyurethane) condoms for either the male or female can be used.

What if I test positive for HIV?

If you test positive for HIV, the sooner you take steps to protect your health, the better. Early medical treatment and a healthy lifestyle can help you stay well. Prompt medical care may delay the onset of AIDS and prevent some life-threatening conditions. There are a number of important steps you can take immediately to protect your health:

- See a licensed health care provider, even if you do not feel sick. Try to find a health care provider who has experience treating HIV. There are now many medications to treat HIV infection and help you maintain your health. It is never too early to start thinking about treatment possibilities.

- Have a TB (tuberculosis) test. You may be infected with TB and not know it. Undetected TB can cause serious illness, but it can be successfully treated if caught early.

- Smoking cigarettes, drinking too much alcohol, or using illegal drugs (such as methamphetamines) can weaken your immune system. There are programs available that can help you stop or reduce your use of these substances.

- Have a screening test for other sexually transmitted diseases (STDs). Undetected STDs can cause serious health problems. It is also important to practice safe-sex behaviors so you can avoid getting STDs.

There is much you can do to stay healthy. Learn all that you can about maintaining good health.

Not having (abstaining from) sex is the most effective way to avoid transmitting HIV to others. If you choose to have sex, use a latex condom to help protect your partner from HIV and other STDs. Studies have shown that latex condoms are very effective, though not 100%, in preventing HIV transmission when used correctly and consistently. If either partner is allergic to latex, plastic (polyurethane) condoms for either the male or female can be used.

I'm HIV positive. Where can I get information about treatments?

CDC recommends that you be in the care of a licensed health care provider, preferably one with experience treating people living with HIV. Your health care provider can assist you with treatment information and guidance.

Why does CDC recommend HIV screening for all pregnant women?

HIV testing during pregnancy is important because antiviral therapy can improve the mother's health and greatly lower the chance of an HIV-infected pregnant woman passing HIV to her infant before, during, or after birth. The treatment is most effective when started as early as possible during pregnancy. CDC recommends HIV screening for all pregnant women because risk-based testing approaches miss many women who are infected with HIV. CDC does recommend providing information on HIV (either orally or by pamphlet) for women with risk factors, as well as referrals to prevention counseling.

HIV testing provides an opportunity for infected women to find out if they are infected and to gain access to medical treatment that may help to delay disease progression. It also allows them to make informed choices that can prevent transmission to their infant. For some women, the prenatal care period could be an ideal opportunity for HIV prevention and subsequent behavior change to reduce risk for acquiring HIV infection

Men on the Down Low

What are the origins of this term down low and what does it refer to?

The most generic definition of the term down low, or DL, is "to keep something private," whether that refers to information or activity.

The term is often used to describe the behavior of men who have sex with other men as well as women and who do not identify as gay or bisexual. These men may refer to themselves as being "on the down low," "on the DL," or "on the low low." The term has most often been associated with African American men. Although the term originated in the African American community, the behaviors associated with the term are not new and not specific to black men who have sex with men.

What are the sexual risk factors associated with being on the down low?

Much of the media attention about men on the down low and HIV/AIDS has focused on the concept of a transmission bridge between bisexual men and heterosexual women. Some women have become infected through sexual contact with bisexual men. However, many questions have not yet been answered, including:

- Do bisexually active men account for more cases of HIV infection in women than do men who inject drugs?

- Are bisexually active men more likely than other groups of men to be HIV infected?

- What proportion of HIV-infected men who have sex with male and female partners identify with the down low?

- Do men on the down low engage in fewer or more sexual risk behaviors than men who are not on the down low?

- Do people other than bisexually active men who do not disclose their behavior to sex partners identify with the down low?

What are the implications for HIV prevention?

The phenomenon of men on the down low has gained much attention in recent years; however, there are no data to confirm or refute publicized accounts of HIV risk behavior associated with these men. What is clear is that women, men, and children of minority races and ethnicities are disproportionately affected by HIV and AIDS and that all persons need to protect themselves and others from getting or transmitting HIV.

What steps is CDC taking to address the down low?

CDC and its many research partners have several projects in the field that are exploring the HIV-related sexual risks of men, including men who use the term down low to refer to themselves. The results of these studies will be published in medical journals and circulated through press releases in the next few years as each study is concluded and the data analyzed. CDC has also funded several projects that provide HIV education, counseling, and testing in minority racial and ethnic communities. CDC's research and on-the-ground HIV prevention efforts will continue as more information about the demographics and HIV risk behaviors of men who do and men who do not identify with the down low becomes available.

How is HIV passed from one person to another?

HIV transmission can occur when blood, semen (cum), pre-seminal fluid (pre-cum), vaginal fluid, or breast milk from an infected person enters the body of an uninfected person.

HIV can enter the body through a vein (e.g., injection drug use), the lining of the anus or rectum, the lining of the vagina and/or cervix, the opening to the penis, the mouth, other mucous membranes (e.g., eyes or inside of the nose), or cuts and sores. Intact, healthy skin is an excellent barrier against HIV and other viruses and bacteria.

These are the most common ways that HIV is transmitted from one person to another:

- by having sex (anal, vaginal, or oral) with an HIV-infected person;
- by sharing needles or injection equipment with an injection drug user who is infected with HIV; or
- from HIV-infected women to their babies before or during birth, or through breast-feeding after birth.

HIV also can be transmitted through receipt of infected blood or blood clotting factors. However, since 1985, all donated blood in the United States has been tested for HIV. Therefore, the risk of infection through transfusion of blood or blood products is extremely low. The U.S. blood supply is considered to be among the safest in the world.

For more information, see *"How safe is the blood supply in the United States?"*)

Some health-care workers have become infected after being stuck with needles containing HIV-infected blood or, less frequently when infected blood comes in contact with a worker's open cut or is splashed into a worker's eyes or inside their nose. There has been only one instance of patients being infected by an HIV-infected dentist to his patients.

Which body fluids transmit HIV?

These body fluids have been shown to contain high concentrations of HIV:

- blood
- semen
- vaginal fluid
- breast milk
- other body fluids containing blood

The following are additional body fluids that may transmit the virus that health care workers may come into contact with:

- fluid surrounding the brain and the spinal cord
- fluid surrounding bone joints
- fluid surrounding an unborn baby

HIV has been found in the saliva and tears of some persons living with HIV, but in very low quantities. It is important to understand that finding a small amount of HIV in a body fluid does not necessarily mean that HIV can be transmitted by that body fluid. HIV has not been recovered from the sweat of HIV-infected persons. Contact with saliva, tears, or sweat has never been shown to result in transmission of HIV.

How well does HIV survive outside the body?

Scientists and medical authorities agree that HIV does not survive well outside the body, making the possibility of environmental transmission remote. HIV is found in varying concentrations or amounts in blood, semen, vaginal fluid, breast milk, saliva, and tears. To obtain data on the survival of HIV, laboratory studies have required the use of artificially high concentrations of laboratory-grown virus. Although these unnatural concentrations of HIV can be kept alive for days or even weeks under precisely controlled and limited laboratory conditions, CDC studies have shown that drying of even these high concentrations of HIV reduces the amount of infectious virus by 90 to 99 percent within several hours. Since the HIV concentrations used in laboratory studies are much higher than those actually found in blood or other specimens, drying of HIV-infected human blood or other body fluids reduces the theoretical risk of environmental transmission to that which has been observed - essentially zero. Incorrect interpretations of conclusions drawn from laboratory studies have in some instances caused unnecessary alarm.

Results from laboratory studies should not be used to assess specific personal risk of infection because (1) the amount of virus studied is not found in human specimens or elsewhere in nature, and (2) no one has been identified as infected with HIV due to contact with an environmental surface. Additionally, HIV is unable to reproduce outside its living host (unlike many bacteria or fungi, which may do so under suitable conditions), except under laboratory conditions; therefore, it does not spread or maintain infectiousness outside its host.

Can I get HIV from kissing?

On the Cheek:

HIV is not transmitted casually, so kissing on the cheek is very safe. Even if the other person has the virus, your unbroken skin is a good barrier. No one has become infected from such ordinary social contact as dry kisses, hugs, and handshakes.

Open-Mouth Kissing:

Open-mouth kissing is considered a very low-risk activity for the transmission of HIV. However, prolonged open-mouth kissing could damage the mouth or lips and allow HIV to pass from an infected person to a partner and then enter the body through cuts or sores in the mouth. Because of this possible risk, the CDC recommends against open-mouth kissing with an infected partner.

One case suggests that a woman became infected with HIV from her sex partner through exposure to contaminated blood during open-mouth kissing.

Can I get HIV from oral sex?

Yes, it is possible for either partner to become infected with HIV through performing or receiving oral sex. There have been a few cases of HIV transmission from performing oral sex on a person infected with HIV. While no one knows exactly what the degree of risk is, evidence suggests that the risk is less than that of unprotected anal or vaginal sex.

If the person performing oral sex has HIV, blood from their mouth may enter the body of the person receiving oral sex through

- the lining of the urethra (the opening at the tip of the penis);
- the lining of the vagina or cervix;
- the lining of the anus; or
- directly into the body through small cuts or open sores.

If the person receiving oral sex has HIV, their blood, semen (cum), pre-seminal fluid (pre-cum), or vaginal fluid may contain the virus. Cells lining the mouth of the person performing oral sex may allow HIV to enter their body.

The risk of HIV transmission increases

- if the person performing oral sex has cuts or sores around or in their mouth or throat;
- if the person receiving oral sex ejaculates in the mouth of the person performing oral sex; or
- if the person receiving oral sex has another sexually transmitted disease (STD).

Not having (abstaining from) sex is the most effective way to avoid HIV.

If you choose to perform oral sex, and your partner is male,

- use a latex condom on the penis; or
- if you or your partner is allergic to latex, plastic (polyurethane) condoms can be used.

Studies have shown that latex condoms are very effective, though not perfect, in preventing HIV transmission when used correctly and consistently. If either partner is allergic to latex, plastic (polyurethane) condoms for either the male or female can be used.

If you choose to have oral sex, and your partner is female,

- use a latex barrier (such as a natural rubber latex sheet, a dental dam or a cut-open condom that makes a square) between your mouth and the vagina. A latex barrier such as a dental dam reduces the risk of blood or vaginal fluids entering your mouth. Plastic food wrap also can be used as a barrier.

If you choose to perform oral sex with either a male or female partner and this sex includes oral contact with your partners anus (analingus or rimming),

- use a latex barrier (such as a natural rubber latex sheet, a dental dam or a cut-open condom that makes a square) between your mouth and the anus. Plastic food wrap also can be used as a barrier.

If you choose to share sex toys with your partner, such as dildos or vibrators,

- each partner should use a new condom on the sex toy; and
- be sure to clean sex toys between each use.

Can I get HIV from anal sex?
Yes. In fact, unprotected (without a condom) anal sex (intercourse) is considered to be very risky behavior. It is possible for either sex partner to become infected with HIV during anal sex. HIV can be found in the blood, semen, pre-seminal fluid, or vaginal fluid of a person infected with the virus. In general, the person receiving the semen is at greater risk of getting HIV because the lining of the rectum is thin and may allow the virus to enter the body during anal sex. However, a person who inserts his penis into an infected partner also is at risk because HIV can enter through the urethra (the opening at the tip of the penis) or through small cuts, abrasions, or open sores on the penis.

Not having (abstaining from) sex is the most effective way to avoid HIV. If people choose to have anal sex, they should use a latex condom. Most of the time, condoms work well. However, condoms are more likely to break during anal sex than during vaginal sex. Thus, even with a condom, anal sex can be risky. A person should use generous amounts of water-based lubricant in addition to the condom to reduce the chances of the condom breaking.

Can I get HIV from vaginal sex*?

Yes, it is possible for either partner to become infected with HIV through vaginal sex* (intercourse). In fact, it is the most common way the virus is transmitted in much of the world. HIV can be found in the blood, semen (cum), pre-seminal fluid (pre-cum) or vaginal fluid of a person infected with the virus.

In women, the lining of the vagina can sometimes tear and possibly allow HIV to enter the body. HIV can also be directly absorbed through the mucous membranes that line the vagina and cervix.

In men, HIV can enter the body through the urethra (the opening at the tip of the penis) or through small cuts or open sores on the penis.

Risk for HIV infection increases if you or a partner has a sexually transmitted disease (STD). See also "Is there a connection between HIV and other sexually transmitted diseases?"

Not having (abstaining from) sex is the most effective way to avoid HIV. If you choose to have vaginal sex, use a latex condom to help protect both you and your partner from HIV and other STDs. Studies have shown that latex condoms are very effective, though not perfect, in preventing HIV transmission when used correctly and consistently. If either partner is allergic to latex, plastic (polyurethane) condoms for either the male or female can be used.

(For the purpose of this FAQ, vaginal sex or intercourse refers to sexual activity between a man and a woman involving the insertion of the penis into the vagina.)

Is there a connection between HIV and other sexually transmitted diseases?

Yes. Having a sexually transmitted disease (STD) can increase a person's risk of becoming infected with HIV, whether the STD causes open sores or breaks in the skin (e.g., syphilis, herpes, chancroid) or does not cause breaks in the skin (e.g., chlamydia, gonorrhea).

If the STD infection causes irritation of the skin, breaks or sores may make it easier for HIV to enter the body during sexual contact. Even when the STD causes no breaks or open sores, the infection can stimulate an immune response in the genital area that can make HIV transmission more likely.

In addition, if an HIV-infected person is also infected with another STD, that person is three to five times more likely than other HIV-infected persons to transmit HIV through sexual contact.

Not having (abstaining from) sexual intercourse is the most effective way to avoid all STDs, including HIV. For those who choose to be sexually active, the following HIV prevention activities are highly effective:

- Engaging in behaviors that do not involve vaginal or anal intercourse or oral sex
- Having sex with only one uninfected partner
- Using latex condoms every time you have sex

Why is injecting drugs a risk for HIV?

At the start of every intravenous injection, blood is introduced into the needle and syringe. HIV can be found in the blood of a person infected with the virus. The reuse of a blood-contaminated needle or syringe by another drug injector (sometimes called "direct syringe sharing") carries a high risk of HIV transmission because infected blood can be injected directly into the bloodstream.

Sharing drug equipment (or "works") can be a risk for spreading HIV. Infected blood can be introduced into drug solutions by

- using blood-contaminated syringes to prepare drugs;

198

- reusing water;
- reusing bottle caps, spoons, or other containers ("spoons" and "cookers") used to dissolve drugs in water and to heat drug solutions; or
- reusing small pieces of cotton or cigarette filters ("cottons") used to filter out particles that could block the needle.

" Street sellers" of syringes may repackage used syringes and sell them as sterile syringes. For this reason, people who continue to inject drugs should obtain syringes from reliable sources of sterile syringes, such as pharmacies.

It is important to know that sharing a needle or syringe for any use, including skin popping and injecting steroids, can put one at risk for HIV and other blood-borne infections.

For more information see "How can injection drug users reduce their risk for HIV infection?"

How can injection drug users reduce their risk for HIV infection?

The CDC recommends that people who inject drugs should be regularly counseled to

- stop using and injecting drugs.
- enter and complete substance abuse treatment, including relapse prevention.
- For injection drug users who cannot or will not stop injecting drugs, the following steps may be taken to reduce personal and public health risks:
- Never reuse or "share" syringes, water, or drug preparation equipment.
- Only use syringes obtained from a reliable source (such as pharmacies or needle exchange programs).
- Use a new, sterile syringe each time to prepare and inject drugs.

- If possible, use sterile water to prepare drugs; otherwise, use clean water from a reliable source (such as fresh tap water).
- Use a new or disinfected container ("cooker") and a new filter ("cotton") to prepare drugs.
- Clean the injection site with a new alcohol swab prior to injection.
- Safely dispose of syringes after one use.

If new, sterile syringes and other drug preparation and injection equipment are not available, then previously used equipment should be boiled in water or disinfected with bleach before reuse

Injection drug users and their sex partners also should take precautions, such as using condoms consistently and correctly, to reduce risks of sexual transmission of HIV. For more information on condoms, see "Male Latex Condoms and Sexually Transmitted Diseases."

Are health care workers at risk of getting HIV on the job?

The risk of health care workers being exposed to HIV on the job is very low, especially if they carefully follow universal precautions (i.e., using protective practices and personal protective equipment to prevent HIV and other blood-borne infections). It is important to remember that casual, everyday contact with an HIV-infected person does not expose health care workers or anyone else to HIV. For health care workers on the job, the main risk of HIV transmission is through accidental injuries from needles and other sharp instruments that may be contaminated with the virus; however even this risk is small. Scientists estimate that the risk of infection from a needle-stick is less than 1 percent, a figure based on the findings of several studies of health care workers who received punctures from HIV-contaminated needles or were otherwise exposed to HIV-contaminated blood.

Although the most important strategy for reducing the risk of occupational HIV transmission is to prevent occupational exposures, plans for postexposure management of health care personnel should be in place.

Are patients in a health care setting at risk of getting HIV?

Although HIV transmission is possible in health care settings, it is extremely rare. Medical experts emphasize that the careful practice of infection control procedures, including universal precautions (i.e., using protective practices and personal protective equipment to prevent HIV and other blood-borne infections), protects patients as well as health care providers from possible HIV transmission in medical and dental offices and hospitals.

For more information on preventing occupational exposure to HIV, refer to the CDC fact sheet, "Preventing Occupational HIV Transmission to Healthcare Personnel" available at http://www.cdc.gov/hiv/pubs/facts/hcwprev.htm.

In 1990, the CDC reported on an HIV-infected dentist in Florida who apparently infected some of his patients while doing dental work. Studies of viral DNA sequences linked the dentist to six of his patients who were also HIV-infected. The CDC has not yet been able to establish how the transmission took place. No additional studies have found any evidence of transmission from provider to patient in health care settings.

CDC has documented rare cases of patients contracting HIV in health care settings from infected donor tissue. Most of these cases occurred due to failures in following universal precautions and infection control guidelines. Most also occurred early in the HIV epidemic, before established screening procedures were in place.

Are "lesbians" or other women who have sex with women at risk for HIV?

Female-to-female transmission of HIV appears to be a rare occurrence. However, there are case reports of female-to-female transmission of HIV. The well documented risk of female-to-male transmission of HIV shows that vaginal secretions and menstrual blood may contain the virus and that mucous membrane (e.g., oral, vaginal) exposure to these secretions has the potential to lead to HIV infection.

In order to reduce the risk of HIV transmission, women who have sex with women should do the following:

- Avoid exposure of a mucous membrane, such as the mouth, (especially non-intact tissue) to vaginal secretions and menstrual blood.

- Use condoms consistently and correctly each and every time for sexual contact with men or when using sex toys. Sex toys should not be shared. No barrier methods for use during oral sex have been evaluated as effective by the FDA. However, natural rubber latex sheets, dental dams, cut open condoms, or plastic wrap may offer some protection from contact with body fluids during oral sex and possibly reduce the risk of HIV transmission.

- Know your own and your partner's HIV status. This knowledge can help uninfected women begin and maintain behavioral changes that reduce the risk of becoming infected. For women who are found to be infected, it can assist in getting early treatment and avoiding infecting others.

Can I get HIV from a bite?

Human Bite:

In 1997, CDC published findings from a state health department investigation of an incident that suggested blood-to-blood transmission of HIV by a human bite. There have been other rare reports in the medical literature in which HIV appeared to have been transmitted by a bite. Severe trauma with extensive tissue tearing and damage and presence of blood were reported in each of these instances. Biting is not a common way of transmitting HIV. In fact, there are numerous reports of bites that did not result in HIV infection.

Non-Human Bite:

HIV is a virus that infects humans and thus cannot be transmitted to or carried by non-human animals. The only exception to this is a few chimpanzees in laboratories that have been artificially infected with HIV. Because HIV is not found in non-human animals it is not possible for HIV to be transmitted from an animal bite, such as from a dog or cat.

Some animals can carry viruses that are similar to HIV, such as FIV (Feline Immunodeficiency Virus) found in cats or SIV (Simian Immunodeficiency Virus) found in apes. These viruses can only exist in their specific animal host and are not transmissible to humans.

Can I get HIV from getting a tattoo or by body piercing?

A risk of HIV transmission does exist if instruments contaminated with blood are either not sterilized or disinfected or are used inappropriately between clients. CDC recommends that instruments that are intended to penetrate the skin be used once, then disposed of or thoroughly cleaned and sterilized between clients.

Personal service workers who do tattooing or body piercing should be educated about how HIV is transmitted and take precautions to prevent transmission of HIV and other blood-borne infections in their settings.

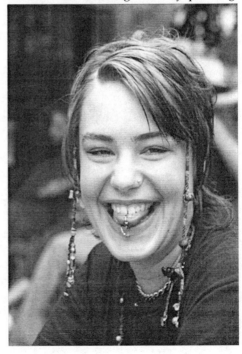

If you are considering getting a tattoo or having your body pierced, ask staff at the establishment what procedures they use to prevent the spread of HIV and other blood-borne infections, such as the hepatitis B virus. You also may call the local health department to find out what sterilization procedures are in place in the local area for these types of establishments.

Can I get HIV from casual contact (shaking hands, hugging, using a toilet, drinking from the same glass, or the sneezing and coughing of an infected person)?

No. HIV is not transmitted by day-to-day contact in the workplace, schools, or social settings. HIV is not transmitted through shaking hands, hugging, or a casual kiss. You cannot become infected from a toilet seat, a drinking fountain, a door knob, dishes, drinking glasses, food, or pets.

HIV is not an airborne or food-borne virus, and it does not live long outside the body. HIV can be found in the blood, semen, or vaginal fluid of an infected person. The three main ways HIV is transmitted are

- through having sex (anal, vaginal, or oral) with someone infected with HIV.
- through sharing needles and syringes with someone who has HIV.
- through exposure (in the case of infants) to HIV before or during birth, or through breast feeding.

Although contact with blood and other body substances can occur in households, transmission of HIV is rare in this setting. A small number of transmission cases have been reported in which a person became infected with HIV as a result of contact with blood or other body secretions from an HIV-infected person in the household. For information on these cases refer to the May 20, 1994 Morbidity and Mortality Weekly Report, "Human Immunodeficiency Virus Transmission in Household Settings — United States"

Persons living with HIV and persons providing home care for those living with HIV should be fully educated and trained regarding appropriate infection-control procedures.

Can I get HIV from mosquitoes?

No. From the start of the HIV epidemic there has been concern about HIV transmission from biting and bloodsucking insects, such as mosquitoes. However, studies conducted by the CDC and elsewhere have shown no evidence of HIV transmission from mosquitoes or any other insects - even in areas where there are many cases of AIDS and large populations of mosquitoes. Lack of such outbreaks, despite intense efforts to detect them, supports the conclusion that HIV is not transmitted by insects.

The results of experiments and observations of insect biting behavior indicate that when an insect bites a person, it does not inject its own or a previously bitten person's or animal's blood into the next person bitten. Rather, it injects saliva, which acts as a lubricant so the insect can feed efficiently. Diseases such as yellow fever and malaria are transmitted through the saliva of specific species of mosquitoes. However, HIV lives for only a short time inside an insect and, unlike organisms that are transmitted via insect bites, HIV does not reproduce (and does not survive) in insects. Thus, even if the virus enters a mosquito or another insect, the insect does not become infected and cannot transmit HIV to the next human it bites.

There also is no reason to fear that a mosquito or other insect could transmit HIV from one person to another through HIV-infected blood left on its mouth parts. Several reasons help explain why this is so. First, infected people do not have constantly high levels of HIV in their blood streams. Second, insect mouth parts retain only very small amounts of blood on their surfaces. Finally, scientists who study insects have determined that biting insects normally do not travel from one person to the next immediately after ingesting blood. Rather, they fly to a resting place to digest the blood meal.

Can I get HIV while playing sports?

There are no documented cases of HIV being transmitted during participation in sports. The very low risk of transmission during sports participation would involve sports with direct body contact in which bleeding might be expected to occur.

If someone is bleeding, their participation in the sport should be interrupted until the wound stops bleeding and is both antiseptically cleaned and securely bandaged. There is no risk of HIV transmission through sports activities where bleeding does not occur.

Frequently Repeated Rumors about HIV Transmission:

I got an e-mail warning that a man, who was believed to be HIV-positive, was recently caught placing blood in the ketchup dispenser at a fast food restaurant. Because of the risk of HIV transmission, the e–mail recommended that only individually wrapped packets of ketchup be used. Is there a risk of contracting HIV from ketchup?

No incidents of ketchup dispensers being contaminated with HIV-infected blood have been reported to CDC. Furthermore, CDC has no reports of HIV infection resulting from eating food, including condiments.

HIV is not an airborne or food-borne virus, and it does not live long outside the body. Even if small amounts of HIV-infected blood were consumed, stomach acid would destroy the virus. Therefore, there is no risk of contracting HIV from eating ketchup.

HIV is most commonly transmitted through specific sexual behaviors (anal, vaginal, or oral sex) or needle sharing with an infected person. An HIV-infected woman can pass the virus to her baby before or during childbirth or after birth through breastfeeding. Although the risk is extremely low in the United Stats, it is also possible to acquire HIV through transfusions of infected blood or blood products.

Did a Texas child die of a heroin overdose after being stuck by a used needle found on a playground?

This story was investigated and found to be a hoax. To become overdosed on a drug from a used needle and syringe, a person would have to have a large amount of the drug injected directly into their body. A needle stick injury such as that mentioned in the story would not lead to a large enough injection to cause a drug overdose. In addition, drug users would leave very little drug material in a discarded syringe after they have injected. If such an incident were to happen, there would likely be concerns about possible blood borne infections, such as human immunodeficiency virus and hepatitis B or C. The risk of these infections from an improperly disposed of needle, such as that described in the story, are extremely low.

Can HIV be transmitted through contact with unused feminine (sanitary) pads?

HIV cannot be transmitted through the use of new, unused feminine pads. The human immunodeficiency virus, or HIV, is a virus that is passed from one person to another through blood-to-blood and sexual contact with someone who is infected with HIV. In addition, infected pregnant women can pass HIV to their babies during pregnancy or delivery, as well as through breast feeding. Although some people have been concerned that HIV might be transmitted in other ways, such as through air, water, insects, or common objects, no scientific evidence supports this. Even though no one has gotten HIV from touching used feminine pads, used pads should be wrapped and properly disposed of so no one comes in contact with blood.

Is a Weekly World News story that claims CDC has discovered a mutated version of HIV that is transmitted through the air true?

This story is not true. It is unfortunate that such stories, which may frighten the public, are being circulated on the Internet.

Human immunodeficiency virus (HIV), the virus that causes AIDS, is spread by sexual contact (anal, vaginal, or oral) or by sharing needles and/or syringes with someone who is infected with HIV.

Babies born to HIV-infected women may become infected before or during birth or through breast feeding.

Many scientific studies have been done to look at all the possible ways that HIV is transmitted. These studies have not shown

HIV to be transmitted through air, water, insects, or casual contact.

I have read stories on the Internet about people getting stuck by needles in phone booth coin returns, movie theater seats, gas pump handles, and other places. One story said that CDC reported similar incidents about improperly discarded needles and syringes. Are these stories true?
CDC has received inquiries about a variety of reports or warnings about used needles left by HIV-infected injection drug users in coin return slots of pay phones, the underside of gas pump handles, and on movie theater seats. These reports and warnings have been circulated on the Internet and by e-mail and fax. Some reports have falsely indicated that CDC "confirmed" the presence of HIV in the needles. CDC has not tested such needles nor has CDC confirmed the presence or absence of HIV in any sample related to these rumors. The majority of these reports and warnings appear to have no foundation in fact.

CDC was informed of one incident in Virginia of a needle stick from a small-gauge needle (believed to be an insulin needle) in a coin return slot of a pay phone. The incident was investigated by the local police department. Several days later, after a report of this police action appeared in the local newspaper, a needle was found in a vending machine but did not cause a needle-stick injury.

Discarded needles are sometimes found in the community outside of health care settings. These needles are believed to have been discarded by persons who use insulin or are injection drug users. Occasionally the "public" and certain groups of workers (e.g., sanitation workers or housekeeping staff) may sustain needle-stick injuries involving inappropriately discarded needles. Needle-stick injuries can transfer blood and blood-borne pathogens (e.g., hepatitis B, hepatitis C, and HIV), but the risk of transmission from discarded needles is extremely low.

CDC does not recommend testing discarded needles to assess the presence or absence of infectious agents in the needles. Management of exposed persons should be done on a case-by-case evaluation of (1) the risk of a blood-borne pathogen infection in the source and (2) the nature of the injury. Anyone who is injured from a needle stick in a community setting should contact their physician or go to an emergency room as soon as possible. The health care professional should then report the injury to the local or state health department. CDC is not aware of any cases where HIV has been transmitted by a needle-stick injury outside a health care setting.

How safe is the blood supply in the United States?

The U.S. blood supply is among the safest in the world. Nearly all people infected with HIV through blood transfusions received those transfusions before 1985, the year HIV testing began for all donated blood.

The Public Health Service has recommended an approach to blood safety in the United States that includes stringent donor selection practices and the use of screening tests. U.S. blood donations have been screened for antibodies to HIV-1 since March 1985 and HIV-2 since June 1992. The p24 Antigen test was added in 1996. Blood and blood products that test positive for HIV are safely discarded and are not used for transfusions.

The improvement of processing methods for blood products also has reduced the number of infections resulting from the use of these products.

Currently, the risk of infection with HIV in the United States through receiving a blood transfusion or blood products is extremely low and has become progressively lower, even in geographic areas with high HIV prevalence rates.

- This list is subject to change as new blood safety opportunities and requirements emerge. Additional tests may be performed to meet special patient needs.

Tests Performed on Each Unit of Donated Blood* (Source: American Red Cross)

Disease	Test	Year Implemented
HIV/ AIDS	HIV/AIDS HIV- I Antibody test	1985
	HIV-1/2 Antibody test	1992
	HIV-I p24 Antigen test	1996
HIV/AIDS and Hepatitis C	Nucleic Acid Test (NAT)	1999
Hepatitis C	Hepatitis C Anti-HCV	1990
Hepatitis B	Hepatitis B Surface Antigen test	1971
	Hepatitis B Core Antibody	1987
Hepatitis	Hepatitis ALT	1986
Syphilis	Syphilis Serologic test	1948
Human T-cell Lymphotropic Virus (HTLV)	HTLV-I Antibody	1989
	HTLV -I/II Antibody	1998

Reference

CDC. HIV/AIDS Surveillance Report, 2003 (Vol. 15). Atlanta: US Department of Health and Human Services, CDC; 2004:1–46.

The Link between HIV and other Sexually Transmitted Infections

Testing and treatment of sexually transmitted diseases (STDs) can be an effective tool in preventing the spread of HIV, the virus that causes AIDS. An understanding of the relationship between STDs and HIV infection can help in the development of effective HIV prevention programs for persons with high-risk sexual behaviors.

Individuals who are infected with STDs are at least two to five times more likely than uninfected individuals to acquire HIV if they are exposed to the virus through sexual contact. In addition, if an HIV-infected individual is also infected with another STD, that person is more likely to transmit HIV through sexual contact than other HIV-infected persons (Wasserheit, 1992).

There is substantial biological evidence demonstrating that the presence of other STDs increases the likelihood of both transmitting and acquiring HIV (Fleming, Wasserheit, 1999).

- Increased susceptibility. STDs probably increase susceptibility to HIV infection by two mechanisms. Genital ulcers (e.g., syphilis, herpes, or chancroid) result in breaks in the genital tract lining or skin. These breaks create a portal of entry for HIV. Non-ulcerative STDs (e.g., chlamydia, gonorrhea, and trichomoniasis) increase the concentration of cells in genital secretions that can serve as targets for HIV (e.g., CD4+ cells).

- Increased infectiousness. Studies have shown that when HIV-infected individuals are also infected with other STDs, they are more likely to have HIV in their genital secretions. For example, men who are infected with both gonorrhea and HIV are more than twice as likely to shed HIV in their genital secretions

211

than are those who are infected only with HIV. Moreover, the median concentration of HIV in semen is as much as 10 times higher in men who are infected with both gonorrhea and HIV than in men infected only with HIV.

Treatment of Other STDs can reduce susceptibility to HIV

Evidence from intervention studies indicates that detecting and treating STDs can substantially reduce HIV transmission at the individual and community levels.

- STD treatment reduces an individual's ability to transmit HIV. Studies have shown that treating STDs in HIV-infected individuals decreases both the amount of HIV they shed and how often they shed the virus (Fleming, Wasserheit, 1999).

- STD treatment reduces the spread of HIV infection in communities. Two community-level, randomized trials have examined the role of STD treatment in HIV transmission. Together, their results have begun to clarify conditions under which STD treatment is likely to be most successful in reducing HIV transmission. First, continuous interventions to improve access to effective STD treatment services are likely to be more effective in reducing HIV transmission than intermittent interventions through strategies such as periodic mass treatment. Second, STD treatment is likely to be most effective in reducing HIV transmission where STD rates are high and the heterosexual HIV epidemic is young. Third, treatment of symptomatic STDs may be particularly important.

- The first community trial, conducted in a rural area of Tanzania, demonstrated a decrease of about 40% in new, heterosexually transmitted HIV infections in communities with continuous access to improved treatment of symptomatic STDs, as compared to communities with minimal STD services, where incidence remained about the same (Grosskurth, Mosha, Todd, et al., 1995). However, in the second trial conducted in Uganda, a reduction in HIV transmission was not demonstrated when the STD control approach was community-wide mass treatment administered to everyone every 10 months in the absence of regular access to improved STD services (Wawer, et al., 1999).

Strong STD prevention, testing, and treatment can play a vital role in comprehensive programs to prevent sexual transmission of HIV. Furthermore, STD trends can offer important insights into where the HIV epidemic may grow, making STD surveillance data helpful in forecasting where HIV rates are likely to increase. Better linkages are needed between HIV and STD prevention efforts nationwide in order to control both epidemics.

In the context of persistently high prevalence of STDs in many parts of the United States and with emerging evidence that the U.S. HIV epidemic increasingly is affecting populations with the highest rates of curable STDs, CDC's Advisory Committee on HIV and STD Prevention (ACHSP) has recommended the following:

- Early detection and treatment of curable STDs should become a major, explicit component of comprehensive HIV prevention programs at national, state, and local levels;

- In areas where STDs that facilitate HIV transmission are prevalent, screening and treatment programs should be expanded;

- HIV and STD prevention programs in the United States, together with private and public sector partners, should take joint responsibility for implementing these strategies.

The ACHSP also notes that early detection and treatment of STDs should be only one component of a comprehensive HIV prevention program, which also must include a range of social, behavioral, and biomedical interventions.

References

Centers for Disease Control and Prevention. 1998. HIV prevention through early detection and treatment of other sexually transmitted diseases - United States. MMWR 47(RR-12):1-24.

Fleming DT, Wasserheit JN. 1999. From epidemiological synergy to public health policy and practice: The contribution of other sexually transmitted diseases to sexual transmission of HIV infection. Sexually Transmitted Infections 75:3-17.

Grosskurth H, Mosha F, Todd J, et al. 1995. Impact of improved treatment of sexually transmitted diseases on HIV infection in rural Tanzania: Randomized controlled trial. Lancet 346:630-6.

Wasserheit JN. 1992. Epidemiologic synergy: Interrelationships between human immunodeficiency virus infection and other sexually transmitted diseases. Sexually Transmitted Diseases 9:61-77.

Wawer MJ, Sewankambo NK, Serwadda D., et al. 1999. Control of sexually transmitted diseases for AIDS prevention in Uganda: a randomized community trial. Rakai Project Study Group. Lancet. 353(9152):525-35.

Coinfection with HIV and Hepatitis C Virus

Overview

Persons with HIV, especially injection drug users, may also be infected with the hepatitis C virus (HCV).

HCV infection is more serious in persons with HIV.

Many persons with HCV don't have any symptoms.

HCV infection can be treated

Injecting drugs is one of the main ways people become infected with HIV. It is also the main way of becoming infected with the hepatitis C virus (HCV). In fact, 50%-90% of HIV-infected injection drug users are also infected with hepatitis C.

HCV infection is more serious in HIV-infected persons.* It leads to liver damage more quickly. Coinfection with HCV may also affect the treatment of HIV infection. Therefore, it's important for HIV-infected persons to know whether they are also infected with HCV and, if they aren't, to take steps to prevent infection.

Many people with hepatitis C don't have any symptoms of the disease. So your doctor or other health care provider will have to test your blood to check for the virus. If you test positive, he or she may also do a liver biopsy to determine the amount of damage to your liver.

Chronic hepatitis C can be treated successfully, even in HIV-infected persons. Treatment for chronic hepatitis C is with a single drug or combination of two drugs. Treatment will usually take 6-12 months. You should drink little or no alcohol during treatment and may be advised not to have alcohol ever again. Vaccination against hepatitis A and hepatitis B is also recommended.

Other Ways of Becoming Infected with HCV

There are other ways of becoming infected with HCV. Persons with hemophilia who received clotting factor concentrates before 1987 commonly have HCV infection. Becoming infected through sexual contact is possible, but the risk is much lower than the risk for HIV. Mothers can pass the infection to their newborn babies, but here too the risk is less than that for HIV.

How to Prevent HCV Infection

The best way to prevent infection with HCV is to stop injecting drugs or never to start. Substance abuse programs may help. If you continue to inject drugs, always use new, sterile syringes and never reuse or share syringes, needles, water or drug preparation equipment. Do not share toothbrushes, razors and other items that might be contaminated with blood. Tattooing or body piercing may also put you at increased risk for infection with any blood-borne pathogen if dirty needles or other instruments are used. Practice safer sex.

Liver Biopsy

During a liver biopsy, a tiny piece of your liver is removed through a needle. The tiny piece (or specimen) is then checked for amount of liver damage.

Treating HCV Infection

Alpha interferon or pegylated interferon alone, or one of these in combination with ribavirin are the drugs given to patients with chronic hepatitis C who are at greatest risk for progression to serious disease. Treatment is not always successful, but even HIV-infected patients may benefit from treatment. Your doctor or other health care provider will need to make the final decision about if and when you should receive treatment.

Reference

Centers for Disease Control and Prevention. Recommendations for prevention and control of hepatitis C virus (HCV) infection and HCV-related chronic disease. MMWR 1998;47(No. RR-19):1-39. Available on the Internet at:

Frequently Asked Questions and Answers About Coinfection with HIV and Hepatitis C Virus

Why should HIV-infected persons be concerned about coinfection with HCV?

About one quarter of HIV-infected persons in the United States are also infected with hepatitis C virus (HCV). HCV is one of the most important causes of chronic liver disease in the United States and HCV infection progresses more rapidly to liver damage in HIV-infected persons. HCV infection may also impact the course and management of HIV infection.

The latest U.S. Public Health Service/Infectious Diseases Society of America (USPHS/IDSA) guidelines recommend that all HIV-infected persons should be screened for HCV infection. Prevention of HCV infection for those not already infected and reducing chronic liver disease in those who are infected are important concerns for HIV-infected individuals and their health care providers.

Who is likely to have HIV-HCV coinfection?

The hepatitis C virus (HCV) is transmitted primarily by large or repeated direct percutaneous (i.e., passage through the skin by puncture) exposures to contaminated blood. Therefore, coinfection with HIV and HCV is common (50%-90%) among HIV-infected injection drug users (IDUs). Coinfection is also common among persons with hemophilia who received clotting factor concentrates before concentrates were effectively treated to inactivate both viruses (i.e., products made before 1987). The risk for acquiring infection through perinatal or sexual exposures is much lower for HCV than for HIV. For persons infected with HIV through sexual exposure (e.g., male-to-male sexual activity), coinfection with HCV is no more common than among similarly aged adults in the general population (3%-5%).

What are the effects of coinfection on disease progression of HCV and HIV?

Chronic HCV infection develops in 75%-85% of infected persons and leads to chronic liver disease in 70% of these chronically infected persons. HIV-HCV coinfection has been associated with higher titers of HCV, more rapid progression to HCV-related liver disease, and an increased risk for HCV-related cirrhosis (scarring) of the liver. Because of this, HCV infection has been viewed as an opportunistic infection in HIV-infected persons and was included in the 1999 USPHS/IDSA Guidelines for the Prevention of Opportunistic Infections in Persons Infected with Human Immunodeficiency Virus. It is not, however, considered an AIDS-defining illness. As highly active antiretroviral therapy (HAART) and prophylaxis of opportunistic infections increase the life span of persons living with HIV, HCV-related liver disease has become a major cause of hospital admissions and deaths among HIV-infected persons.

The effects of HCV coinfection on HIV disease progression are less certain. Some studies have suggested that infection with certain HCV genotypes is associated with more rapid progression to AIDS or death. However, the subject remains controversial. Since coinfected patients are living longer on HAART, more data are needed to determine if HCV infection influences the long-term natural history of HIV infection.

How can coinfection with HCV be prevented?

Persons living with HIV who are not already coinfected with HCV can adopt measures to prevent acquiring HCV. Such measures will also reduce the chance of transmitting their HIV infection to others.

Not injecting or stopping injection drug use would eliminate the chief route of HCV transmission; substance-abuse treatment and relapse-prevention programs should be recommended. If patients continue to inject, they should be counseled about safer injection practices; that is, to use new, sterile syringes every time they inject drugs and never reuse or share syringes, needles, water, or drug preparation equipment.

Toothbrushes, razors, and other personal care items that might be contaminated with blood should not be shared. Although there are no data from the United States indicating that tattooing and body piercing place persons at increased risk for HCV infection, these procedures may be a source for infection with any bloodborne pathogen if proper infection control practices are not followed.

Although consistent data are lacking regarding the extent to which sexual activity contributes to HCV transmission, persons having multiple sex partners are at risk for other sexually transmitted diseases (STDs) as well as for transmitting HIV to others. They should be counseled accordingly.

How should patients coinfected with HIV and HCV be managed?

General guidelines

Patients coinfected with HIV and HCV should be encouraged to adopt safe behaviors (as described in the previous section) to prevent transmission of HIV and HCV to others.

Individuals with evidence of HCV infection should be given information about prevention of liver damage, undergo evaluation for chronic liver disease and, if indicated, be considered for treatment. Persons coinfected with HIV and HCV should be advised not to drink excessive amounts of alcohol. Avoiding alcohol altogether might be wise because the effects of even moderate or low amounts of alcohol (e.g., 12 oz. of beer, 5 oz. of wine or 1.5 oz. hard liquor per day) on disease progression are unknown. When appropriate, referral should be made to alcohol treatment and relapse-prevention programs. Because of possible effects on the liver, HCV- infected patients should consult with their health care professional before taking any new medicines, including over-the-counter, alternative or herbal medicines.

Susceptible coinfected patients should receive hepatitis A vaccine because the risk for fulminant hepatitis associated with hepatitis A is increased in persons with chronic liver disease. Susceptible patients should receive hepatitis B vaccine because most HIV-infected persons are at risk for HBV infection. The vaccines appear safe for these patients and more than two-thirds of those vaccinated develop antibody responses. Prevaccination screening for antibodies against hepatitis A and hepatitis B in this high-prevalence population is generally cost-effective. Postvaccination testing for hepatitis A is not recommended, but testing for antibody to hepatitis B surface antigen (anti-HBs) should be performed 1-2 months after completion of the primary series of hepatitis B vaccine. Persons who fail to respond should be revaccinated with up to three additional doses.

HAART has no significant effect on HCV. However, coinfected persons may be at increased risk for HAART-associated liver toxicity and should be closely monitored during antiretroviral therapy. Data suggest that the majority of these persons do not appear to develop significant and/or symptomatic hepatitis after initiation of antiretroviral therapy.

Treatment for HCV Infection

A Consensus Development Conference Panel convened by The National Institutes of Health in 1997 recommended antiviral therapy for patients with chronic hepatitis C who are at the greatest risk for progression to cirrhosis. These persons include anti-HCV positive patients with persistently elevated liver enzymes, detectable HCV RNA, and a liver biopsy that indicates either portal or bridging fibrosis or at least moderate degrees of inflammation and necrosis. Patients with less severe histological disease should be managed on an individual basis.

In the United States, two different regimens have been approved as therapy for chronic hepatitis C: monotherapy with alpha interferon and combination therapy with alpha interferon and ribavirin. Among HIV-negative persons with chronic hepatitis C, combination therapy consistently yields higher rates (30%-40%) of sustained response than monotherapy (10%-20%). Combination therapy is more effective against viral genotypes 2 and 3, and requires a shorter course of treatment; however, viral genotype 1 is the most common among U.S. patients. Combination therapy is associated with more side effects than monotherapy, but, in most situations, it is preferable. At present, interferon monotherapy is reserved for patients who have contraindications to the use of ribavirin.

Studies thus far, although not extensive, have indicated that response rates in HIV-infected patients to alpha interferon monotherapy for HCV were lower than in non-HIV-infected patients, but the differences were not statistically significant. Monotherapy appears to be reasonably well tolerated in coinfected patients. There are no published articles on the long-term effect of combination therapy in coinfected patients, but studies currently underway suggest it is superior to monotherapy. However, the side effects of combination therapy are greater in coinfected patients. Thus, combination therapy should be used with caution until more data are available.

220

The decision to treat people coinfected with HIV and HCV must also take into consideration their concurrent medications and medical conditions. If CD4 counts are normal or minimally abnormal (> 400/ul), there is little difference in treatment success rates between those who are coinfected and those who are infected with HCV alone.

Other Treatment Considerations

Persons with chronic hepatitis C who continue to abuse alcohol are at risk for ongoing liver injury, and antiviral therapy may be ineffective. Therefore, strict abstinence from alcohol is recommended during antiviral therapy, and interferon should be given with caution to a patient who has only recently stopped alcohol abuse. Typically, a 6-month abstinence is recommended for alcohol abusers before starting therapy; such patients should be treated with the support and collaboration of alcohol abuse treatment programs.

Although there is limited experience with antiviral treatment for chronic hepatitis C of persons who are recovering from long-term injection drug use, there are concerns that interferon therapy could be associated with relapse into drug use, both because of its side effects and because it is administered by injection. There is even less experience with treatment of persons who are active injection drug users, and an additional concern for this group is the risk for reinfection with HCV. Although a 6-month abstinence before starting therapy also has been recommended for injection drug users, additional research is needed on the benefits and drawbacks of treating these patients. Regardless, when patients with past or continuing problems of substance abuse are being considered for treatment, such patients should be treated only in collaboration with substance abuse specialists or counselors. Patients can be successfully treated while on methadone maintenance treatment of addiction.

Because many coinfected patients have conditions or factors (such as major depression or active illicit drug or alcohol use) that may prevent or complicate antiviral therapy, treatment for chronic hepatitis C in HIV-infected patients should be coordinated by health care providers with experience in treating coinfected patients or in clinical trials. It is not known if maintenance therapy is needed after successful therapy, but patients should be counseled to avoid injection drug use and other behaviors that could lead to reinfection with HCV and should continue to abstain from alcohol.

Infections in Infants and Children

The average rate of HCV infection among infants born to women coinfected with HCV and HIV is 14% to 17%, higher than among infants born to women infected with HCV alone. Data are limited on the natural history of HCV infection in children, and antiviral drugs for chronic hepatitis C are not FDA-approved for use in children under aged 18 years. Therefore, children should be referred to a pediatric hepatologist or similar specialist for management and for determination for eligibility in clinical trials.

What research is needed on HIV-HCV coinfection?

Many important questions remain about HIV-HCV coinfection:

By what mechanism does HIV infection affect the natural history of hepatitis C?

Does HAART affect the impact of HIV on the natural history of HCV infection?

Does HCV affect the natural history of HIV and, if so, by what mechanism?

How can we effectively and safely treat chronic hepatitis C in HIV-infected patients?

How can we distinguish between liver toxicity caused by antiretrovirals and that caused by HCV infection?

What is the best protocol for treating both HIV and chronic hepatitis C in the coinfected patient?

The Deadly Intersection between TB and HIV

Tuberculosis (TB) is a disease that is spread from person-to-person through the air, and it is particularly dangerous for people infected with HIV. Worldwide, TB is the leading cause of death among people infected with HIV.

An estimated 10-15 million Americans are infected with TB bacteria, with the potential to develop active TB disease in the future. About 10 percent of these infected individuals will develop TB at some point in their lives. However, the risk of developing TB disease is much greater for those infected with HIV and living with AIDS. Because HIV infection so severely weakens the immune system, people dually infected with HIV and TB have a 100 times greater risk of developing active TB disease and becoming infectious compared to people not infected with HIV. CDC estimates that 10 to 15 percent of all TB cases and nearly 30 percent of cases among people ages 25 to 44 are occurring in HIV-infected individuals.

This high level of risk underscores the critical need for targeted TB screening and preventive treatment programs for HIV-infected people and those at greatest risk for HIV infection. All people infected with HIV should be tested for TB, and, if infected, complete preventive therapy as soon as possible to prevent TB disease.

Intersection of Two Global Epidemics

- Approximately 2 billion people (one-third of the world's population) are infected with Mycobacterium tuberculosis, the cause of TB.

- TB is the cause of death for one out of every three people with AIDS worldwide.

- The spread of the HIV epidemic has significantly impacted the TB epidemic - one-third of the increase in TB cases over the last five years can be attributed to the HIV epidemic (Source: UNAIDS).

The Continued Threat of Multidrug-Resistant TB

Every nation must face the challenge of combating multidrug-resistant (MDR) TB. People infected with HIV and living with AIDS are at greater risk for developing MDR TB. MDR TB is extremely difficult to treat and can be fatal. While the number of cases has remained stable in the United States over the past few years, people with MDR TB have now been reported from 43 states and the District of Columbia.

To prevent the continued emergence of drug-resistant strains of TB, treatment for TB must be improved in the United States and across the globe. Inconsistent or partial treatment is the main cause of TB that is resistant to available drugs (MDR-TB.) The most effective strategy for ensuring completion of treatment is Directly Observed Therapy, and its use must be expanded.

Another challenge that individuals co-infected with HIV and TB face is the possible complications that can occur when taking HIV treatment regimens along with drugs commonly used to treat TB. Physicians prescribing these drugs must carefully consider all potential interactions.

Addressing the Dangers of the Interconnected TB/HIV Epidemics Requires Expanded Efforts

TB control is an exercise in vigilance; the goal of controlling and eventually eliminating TB requires a targeted and continuous effort to address the prevention and treatment needs for those most at risk, including HIV-infected individuals. Efforts to eliminate TB are therefore essential to reducing the global toll of HIV.

Cytomegalovirus (CMV) Infection

Cytomegalovirus, or CMV, is found universally throughout all geographic locations and socioeconomic groups, and infects between 50% and 85% of adults in the United States by 40 years of age. CMV is also the virus most frequently transmitted to a developing child before birth. CMV infection is more widespread in developing countries and in areas of lower socioeconomic conditions. For most healthy persons *who acquire CMV after birth* there are few symptoms and no long-term health consequences. Some persons with symptoms experience a mononucleosis-like syndrome with prolonged fever, and a mild hepatitis. Once a person becomes infected, the virus remains alive, but usually dormant within that person's body for life. Recurrent disease rarely occurs unless the person's immune system is suppressed due to therapeutic drugs or disease. Therefore, for the vast majority of people, CMV infection is not a serious problem.

However, CMV infection is important to certain high-risk groups. Major areas of concern are:

- the risk of infection to the unborn baby during pregnancy,
- the risk of infection to people who work with children, and
- the risk of infection to the immunocompromised person, such as organ transplant recipients and persons infected with human immunodeficiency virus (HIV).

CMV is a member of the herpesvirus group, which includes herpes simplex virus types 1 and 2, varicella-zoster virus (which causes chickenpox), and Epstein-Barr virus (which causes infectious mononucleosis). These viruses share a characteristic ability to remain dormant within the body over a long period. Initial CMV infection, which may have few symptoms, is always followed by a prolonged, inapparent infection during which the vi-

225

rus resides in cells without causing detectable damage or clinical illness. Severe impairment of the body's immune system by medication or disease consistently reactivates the virus from the latent or dormant state.

Infectious CMV may be shed in the bodily fluids of any previously infected person, and thus may be found in urine, saliva, blood, tears, semen, and breast milk. The shedding of virus may take place intermittently, without any detectable signs, and without causing symptoms.

Prevention

Transmission of CMV occurs from person to person. Infection requires close, intimate contact with a person excreting the virus in their saliva, urine, or other bodily fluids. CMV can be sexually transmitted and can also be transmitted via breast milk, transplanted organs, and rarely from blood transfusions.

Although the virus is not highly contagious, it has been shown to spread in households and among young children in day care centers. Transmission of the virus is often preventable because it is most often transmitted through infected bodily fluids that come in contact with hands and then are absorbed through the nose or mouth of a susceptible person. Therefore, care should be taken when handling children and items like diapers. Simple hand washing with soap and water is effective in removing the virus from the hands.

CMV infection without symptoms is common in infants and young children; therefore, it is unjustified and unnecessary to exclude from school or an institution a child known to be infected. Similarly, hospitalized patients do not need separate or elaborate isolation precautions.

Screening children and patients for CMV is of questionable value. The cost and management of such procedures are impractical. Children known to have CMV infection should not be singled out for exclusion, isolation, or special handling. Instead, staff education and effective hygiene practices are advised in caring for all children.

CIRCUMSTANCES IN WHICH CMV INFECTION COULD BE A PROBLEM

Pregnancy

The incidence of primary (or first) CMV infection in pregnant women in the United States varies from 1% to 3%. Healthy pregnant women are not at special risk for disease from CMV infection. When infected with CMV, most women have no symptoms and very few have a disease resembling mononucleosis. It is their developing unborn babies that may be at risk for congenital CMV disease. CMV remains the most important cause of congenital (meaning from birth) viral infection in the United States. For infants who are infected by their mothers before birth, two potential problems exist:

- Generalized infection may occur in the infant, and symptoms may range from moderate enlargement of the liver and spleen (with jaundice) to fatal illness. With supportive treatment most infants with CMV disease usually survive. However, from 80% to 90% will have complications within the first few years of life that may include hearing loss, vision impairment, and varying degrees of mental retardation.

- Another 5% to 10% of infants who are infected but without symptoms at birth will subsequently have varying degrees of hearing and mental or coordination problems.

However, these risks appear to be *almost exclusively associated* with women who previously have not been infected with CMV and who are having *their first infection* with the virus during pregnancy. Even in this case, two-thirds of the infants will not become infected, and only 10% to 15% of the remaining third will have symptoms at the time of birth. There appears to be little risk of CMV-related complications for women who have been infected at least 6 months prior to conception. For this group, which makes up 50% to 80% of the women of child-bearing age, the rate of newborn CMV infection is 1%, and these infants appear to have no significant illness or abnormalities.

227

The virus can also be transmitted to the infant at delivery from contact with genital secretions or later in infancy through breast milk. However, these infections usually result in little or no clinical illness in the infant.

To summarize, during a pregnancy when a woman *who has never had CMV infection* becomes infected with CMV, there is a potential risk that after birth the infant may have CMV-related complications, the most common of which are associated with hearing loss, visual impairment, or diminished mental and motor capabilities. On the other hand, infants and children *who acquire CMV after birth* have few, if any, symptoms or complications.

Recommendations for pregnant women with regard to CMV infection:

- Throughout the pregnancy, practice good personal hygiene, especially handwashing with soap and water, after contact with diapers or oral secretions (particularly with a child who is in day care).

- Women who develop a mononucleosis-like illness during pregnancy should be evaluated for CMV infection and counseled about the possible risks to the unborn child.

- Laboratory testing for antibody to CMV can be performed to determine if a women has already had CMV infection.

- Recovery of CMV from the cervix or urine of women at or before the time of delivery does not warrant a cesarean section.

- The demonstrated benefits of breast-feeding outweigh the minimal risk of acquiring CMV from the breast-breeding mother.

- There is no need to either screen for CMV or exclude CMV-excreting children from schools or institutions because the virus is frequently found in many healthy children and adults.

People Who Work with Infants and Children

Most healthy people working with infants and children face no special risk from CMV infection. However, for women of child-bearing age who previously have not been infected with CMV, there is a potential risk to the developing unborn child (the risk is described above in the Pregnancy section). Contact with children who are in day care, where CMV infection is commonly transmitted among young children (particularly toddlers), may be a source of exposure to CMV. Since CMV is transmitted through contact with infected body fluids, including urine and saliva, child care providers (meaning day care workers, special education teachers, therapists, as well as mothers) should be educated about the risks of CMV infection and the precautions they can take. Day care workers appear to be at a greater risk than hospital and other health care providers, and this may be due in part to the increased emphasis on personal hygiene in the health care setting.

Recommendations for individuals providing care for infants and children:

- Female employees should be educated concerning CMV, its transmission, and hygienic practices, such as handwashing, which minimize the risk of infection.

- Susceptible nonpregnant women working with infants and children should not routinely be transferred to other work situations.

- Pregnant women working with infants and children should be informed of the risk of acquiring CMV infection and the possible effects on the unborn child.

- Routine laboratory testing for CMV antibody in female workers is not recommended, but can be performed to determine their immune status.

Immunocompromised Patients

Primary (or the initial) CMV infection in the immunocompromised patient can cause serious disease. However, the more common problem is the reactivation of the dormant virus. Infection with CMV is a major cause of disease and death in immunocompromised patients, including organ transplant recipients, patients undergoing hemodialysis, patients with cancer, patients receiving immunosuppressive drugs, and HIV-infected patients. Pneumonia, retinitis (an infection of the eyes), and gastrointestinal disease are the common manifestations of disease. Because of this risk, exposing immunosuppressed patients to outside sources of CMV should be minimized. Whenever possible, patients without CMV infection should be given organs and/or blood products that are free of the virus.

Diagnosis

Most infections with CMV are not diagnosed because the virus usually produces few, if any, symptoms and tends to reactivate intermittently without symptoms. However, persons who have been infected with CMV develop antibodies to the virus, and these antibodies persist in the body for the lifetime of that individual. A number of laboratory tests that detect these antibodies to CMV have been developed to determine if infection has occurred and are widely available from commercial laboratories. In addition, the virus can be cultured from specimens obtained from urine, throat swabs, and tissue samples to detect active infection.

CMV should be suspected if a patient:

- has symptoms of infectious mononucleosis but has negative test results for mononucleosis and Epstein Barr virus, or,
- shows signs of hepatitis, but has negative test results for hepatitis A, B, and C.

For best diagnostic results, laboratory tests for CMV antibody should be performed by using paired serum samples. One blood sample should be taken upon suspicion of CMV, and another one taken within 2 weeks. A virus culture can be performed at any time the patient is symptomatic.

Laboratory testing for antibody to CMV can be performed to determine if a woman has already had CMV infection. However, routine laboratory testing of all pregnant women is costly and the need for testing should therefore be evaluated on a case-by-case basis.

Serologic Testing

The enzyme-linked immunosorbent assay (or ELISA) is the most commonly available serologic test for measuring antibody to CMV. The result can be used to determine if acute infection, prior infection, or passively acquired maternal antibody in an infant is present. Other tests include various fluorescence assays, indirect hemagglutination, and latex agglutination.

An ELISA technique for CMV-specific IgM is available, but may give false-positive results unless steps are taken to remove rheumatoid factor or most of the IgG antibody before the serum sample is tested. Because CMV-specific IgM may be produced in low levels in reactivated CMV infection, its presence is not always indicative of primary infection. Only virus recovered from a target organ, such as the lung, provides unequivocal evidence that the current illness is caused by *acquired CMV infection*. If serologic tests detect a positive or high titer of IgG, this result should not automatically be interpreted to mean that active CMV infection is present. However, if antibody tests of paired serum samples show a fourfold rise in IgG antibody and a significant level of IgM antibody, meaning equal to at least 30% of the IgG value, or virus is cultured from a urine or throat specimen, the findings indicate that an active CMV infection is present.

Treatment

Currently, no treatment exists for CMV infection in the healthy individual. Antiviral drug therapy is now being evaluated in infants. Ganciclovir treatment is used for patients with depressed immunity who have either sight-related or life-threatening illnesses. Vaccines are still in the research and development stage.

Birth Control Methods and Protection against STDs

The Food and Drug Administration has approved a number of birth control methods, ranging from over-the-counter male and female condoms and vaginal spermicides to doctor-prescribed birth control pills, diaphragms, intrauterine devices (IUDs), injected hormones, and hormonal implants. Other contraceptive options include fertility awareness and voluntary surgical sterilization.

The choice of birth control depends on factors such as a person's health, frequency of sexual activity, number of partners, and desire to have children in the future. Effectiveness rates, based on statistical estimates, are another key consideration.

Barrier Methods

Male Condom.

The male condom is a sheath placed over the erect penis before penetration, preventing pregnancy by blocking the passage of sperm.

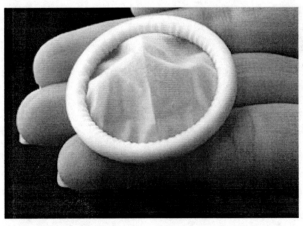

A condom can be used only once. Some have spermicide added, usually nonoxynol-9 in the United States, to kill sperm. Spermicide has not been scientifically shown to provide additional contraceptive protection over the condom alone. Because they act as a mechanical barrier, condoms prevent direct vaginal contact with semen, infectious genital secretions, and genital lesions and discharges.

Most condoms are made from latex rubber, while a small percentage are made from lamb intestines (sometimes called "lambskin" condoms). Condoms made from polyurethane have been marketed in the United States since 1994.

Except for abstinence, latex condoms are the most effective method for reducing the risk of infection from the viruses that cause AIDS, other HIV-related illnesses, and other STDs.

Some condoms are prelubricated. These lubricants don't provide more birth control or STD protection. Non-oil-based lubricants, such as water or K-Y jelly, can be used with latex or lambskin condoms, but oil-based lubricants, such as petroleum jelly (Vaseline), lotions, or massage or baby oil, should not be used because they can weaken the material.

Female condom.

The Reality Female Condom, approved by FDA in April 1993, consists of a lubricated polyurethane sheath shaped similarly to

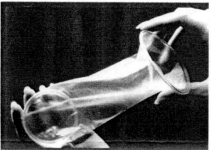

the male condom. The closed end, which has a flexible ring, is inserted into the vagina, while the open end remains outside, partially covering the labia.

The female condom, like the male condom, is available without a prescription and is intended for one-time use. It should not be used together with a male condom because they may not both stay in place.

234

Insertion of Female Condom

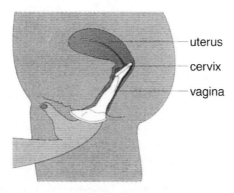

uterus

cervix

vagina

Diaphragm.

Available by prescription only and sized by a health professional to achieve a proper fit, the diaphragm has a dual mechanism to prevent pregnancy. A dome-shaped rubber disk with a flexible rim covers the cervix so sperm can't reach the uterus, while a spermicide applied to the diaphragm before insertion kills sperm.

The diaphragm protects for six hours. For intercourse after the six-hour period, or for repeated intercourse within this period, fresh spermicide should be placed in the vagina with the diaphragm still in place. The diaphragm should be left in place for at least six hours after the last intercourse but not for longer than a total of 24 hours because of the risk of toxic shock syndrome (TSS), a rare but potentially fatal infection. Symptoms of TSS include sudden fever, stomach upset, sunburn-like rash, and a drop in blood pressure.

Cervical cap.

The cap is a soft rubber cup with a round rim, sized by a health professional to fit snugly around the cervix. It is available by prescription only and, like the diaphragm, is used with spermicide.

It protects for 48 hours and for multiple acts of intercourse within this time. Wearing it for more than 48 hours is not recommended because of the risk, though low, of TSS. Also, with prolonged use of two or more days, the cap may cause an unpleasant vaginal odor or discharge in some women.

Sponge.

The vaginal contraceptive sponge has not been available since the sole manufacturer, Whitehall Laboratories of Madison, N.J., voluntarily stopped selling it in 1995. It remains an approved product and could be marketed again.

The sponge, a donut-shaped polyurethane device containing the spermicide nonoxynol-9, is inserted into the vagina to cover the cervix. A woven polyester loop is designed to ease removal.

The sponge protects for up to 24 hours and for multiple acts of intercourse within this time. It should be left in place for at least six hours after intercourse but should be removed no more than 30 hours after insertion because of the risk, though low, of TSS.

Vaginal Spermicides Alone

Vaginal spermicides are available in foam, cream, jelly, film, suppository, or tablet forms. All types contain a sperm-killing chemical.

Studies have not produced definitive data on the efficacy of spermicides alone, but according to the authors of Contraceptive Technology, a leading resource for contraceptive information, the failure rate for typical users may be 21 percent per year.

Package instructions must be carefully followed because some spermicide products require the couple to wait 10 minutes or more after inserting the spermicide before having sex. One dose of spermicide is usually effective for one hour. For repeated intercourse, additional spermicide must be applied. And after intercourse, the spermicide has to remain in place for at least six to eight hours to ensure that all sperm are killed. The woman should not douche or rinse the vagina during this time.

Hormonal Methods

Combined oral contraceptives.

Typically called "the pill," combined oral contraceptives have been on the market for more than 35 years and are the most popular form of reversible birth control in the United States. This form of birth control suppresses ovulation (the monthly release of an egg from the ovaries) by the combined actions of the hormones estrogen and progestin.

If a woman remembers to take the pill every day as directed, she has an extremely low chance of becoming pregnant in a year. But the pill's effectiveness may be reduced if the woman is taking some medications, such as certain antibiotics.

Besides preventing pregnancy, the pill offers additional benefits. As stated in the labeling, the pill can make periods more regular. It also has a protective effect against pelvic inflammatory disease, an infection of the fallopian tubes or uterus that is a major cause of infertility in women, and against ovarian and endometrial cancers.

The decision whether to take the pill should be made in consultation with a health professional. Birth control pills are safe for most women--safer even than delivering a baby--but they carry some risks.

Current low-dose pills have fewer risks associated with them than earlier versions. But women who smoke--especially those over 35--and women with certain medical conditions, such as a history of blood clots or breast or endometrial cancer, may be advised against taking the pill. The pill may contribute to cardiovascular disease, including high blood pressure, blood clots, and blockage of the arteries.

One of the biggest questions has been whether the pill increases the risk of breast cancer in past and current pill users. An international study published in the September 1996 journal Contraception concluded that women's risk of breast cancer 10 years after going off birth control pills was no higher than that of women who had never used the pill. During pill use and for the first 10 years after stopping the pill, women's risk of breast cancer was only slightly higher in pill users than non-pill users.

Side effects of the pill, which often subside after a few months' use, include nausea, headache, breast tenderness, weight gain, irregular bleeding, and depression.

Doctors sometimes prescribe higher doses of combined oral contraceptives for use as "morning after" pills to be taken within 72 hours of unprotected intercourse to prevent the possibly fertilized egg from reaching the uterus. On June 28, 1996, FDA's Advisory Committee for Reproductive Health Drugs concluded that certain oral contraceptives are safe and effective for this use. At press time in January, no drug firm had submitted an application to FDA to label its pills for this use, and the agency had not yet acted on the committee's recommendation.

Minipills.

Although taken daily like combined oral contraceptives, minipills contain only the hormone progestin and no estrogen. They work by reducing and thickening cervical mucus to prevent sperm from reaching the egg. They also keep the uterine lining from thickening, which prevents a fertilized egg from implanting in the uterus. These pills are slightly less effective than combined oral contraceptives.

Minipills can decrease menstrual bleeding and cramps, as well as the risk of endometrial and ovarian cancer and pelvic inflammatory disease. Because they contain no estrogen, minipills don't present the risk of blood clots associated with estrogen in combined pills. They are a good option for women who can't take estrogen because they are breast-feeding or because estrogen-containing products cause them to have severe headaches or high blood pressure.

Side effects of minipills include menstrual cycle changes, weight gain, and breast tenderness.

Injectable progestins.

Depo-Provera, approved by FDA in 1992, is injected by a health professional into the buttocks or arm muscle every three months. Depo-Provera prevents pregnancy in three ways: It inhibits ovulation, changes the cervical mucus to help prevent sperm from reaching the egg, and changes the uterine lining to prevent the fertilized egg from implanting in the uterus. The progestin injection is extremely effective in preventing pregnancy, in large part because it requires little effort for the woman to comply: She simply has to get an injection by a doctor once every three months.

The benefits are similar to those of the minipill and another progestin-only contraceptive, Norplant. Side effects are also similar and can include irregular or missed periods, weight gain, and breast tenderness.

Implantable progestins.

Norplant, approved by FDA in 1990, and the newer Norplant 2, approved in 1996, are the third type of progestin-only contraceptive. Made up of matchstick-sized rubber rods, this contraceptive is surgically implanted under the skin of the upper arm, where it steadily releases the contraceptive steroid levonorgestrel.

The six-rod Norplant provides protection for up to five years (or until it is removed), while the two-rod Norplant 2 protects for up to three years. Norplant failures are rare, but are higher with increased body weight.

Some women may experience inflammation or infection at the site of the implant. Other side effects include menstrual cycle changes, weight gain, and breast tenderness.

Intrauterine Devices

An IUD is a T-shaped device inserted into the uterus by a health-care professional. Two types of IUDs are available in the United States: the Paragard CopperT 380A and the Progestasert Progesterone T. The Paragard IUD can remain in place for 10 years, while the Progestasert IUD must be replaced every year.

It's not entirely clear how IUDs prevent pregnancy. They seem to prevent sperm and eggs from meeting by either immobilizing the sperm on their way to the fallopian tubes or changing the uterine lining so the fertilized egg cannot implant in it.

IUDs have one of the lowest failure rates of any contraceptive method. "In the population for which the IUD is appropriate--for those in a mutually monogamous, stable relationship who aren't at a high risk of infection--the IUD is a very safe and very effective method of contraception," says Lisa Rarick, M.D., director of FDA's division of reproductive and urologic drug products.

IUD in Position

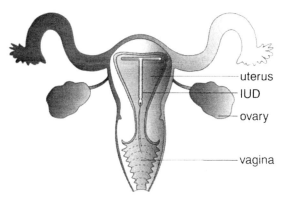

The IUD's image suffered when the Dalkon Shield IUD was taken off the market in 1975. This IUD was associated with a high incidence of pelvic infections and infertility, and some deaths. Today, serious complications from IUDs are rare, although IUD users may be at increased risk of developing pelvic inflammatory disease. Other side effects can include perforation of the uterus, abnormal bleeding, and cramps. Complications occur most often during and immediately after insertion.

Traditional Methods

Fertility awareness.

Also known as natural family planning or periodic abstinence, fertility awareness entails not having sexual intercourse on the days of a woman's menstrual cycle when she could become pregnant or using a barrier method of birth control on those days.

Because a sperm may live in the female's reproductive tract for up to seven days and the egg remains fertile for about 24 hours, a woman can get pregnant within a substantial window of time--from seven days before ovulation to three days after. Methods to approximate when a woman is fertile are usually based on the menstrual cycle, changes in cervical mucus, or changes in body temperature.

"Natural family planning can work," Rarick says, "but it takes an extremely motivated couple to use the method effectively."

Withdrawal.

In this method, also called coitus interruptus, the man withdraws his penis from the vagina before ejaculation. Fertilization is prevented because the sperm don't enter the vagina.

Effectiveness depends on the male's ability to withdraw before ejaculation. Also, withdrawal doesn't provide protection from STDs, including HIV. Infectious diseases can be transmitted by direct contact with surface lesions and by pre-ejaculatory fluid.

Surgical Sterilization

Surgical sterilization is a contraceptive option intended for people who don't want children in the future. It is considered permanent because reversal requires major surgery that is often unsuccessful.

Female sterilization.

Female sterilization blocks the fallopian tubes so the egg can't travel to the uterus. Sterilization is done by various surgical techniques, usually under general anesthesia.

Complications from these operations are rare and can include infection, hemorrhage, and problems related to the use of general anesthesia.

Male sterilization.

This procedure, called a vasectomy, involves sealing, tying or cutting a man's vas deferens, which otherwise would carry the sperm from the testicle to the penis.

Vasectomy involves a quick operation, usually less than 30 minutes, with possible minor postsurgical complications, such as bleeding or infection.

Research continues on effective contraceptives that minimize side effects. One important research focus, according to FDA's Rarick, is the development of birth control methods that are both spermicidal and microbicidal to prevent not only pregnancy but also transmission of HIV and other STDs.

Some people mistakenly believe that by protecting themselves against pregnancy, they are automatically protecting themselves from HIV, the virus that causes AIDS, and other sexually transmitted diseases (STDs). But the male latex condom is the only contraceptive method considered highly effective in reducing the risk of STDs.

Unlike latex condoms, lambskin condoms are not recommended for STD prevention because they are porous and may permit passage of viruses like HIV, hepatitis B and herpes. Polyurethane condoms are an alternative method of STD protection for those who are latex-sensitive.

Because it is a barrier method that works in much the same way as the male condom, the female condom may provide some protection against STDs. Both condoms should not be used together, however, because they may not both stay in place.

According to an FDA advisory committee panel that met Nov. 22, 1996, it appears, based on several published scientific studies, that some vaginal spermicides containing nonoxynol-9 may reduce the risk of gonorrhea and chlamydia transmission. However, use of nonoxynol-9 may cause tissue irritation, raising the possibility of an increased susceptibility to some STDs, including HIV.

As stated in their labeling, birth control pills, Norplant, Depo-Provera, IUDs, and lambskin condoms do not protect against STD infection. For STD protection, a male latex condom can be used in combination with non-condom methods. The relationship of the vaginal barrier methods--the diaphragm, cap and sponge--to STD prevention is not yet clear.

Efficacy rates in this chart are based on Contraceptive Technology (16th edition, 1994). They are yearly estimates of effectiveness in typical use, which refers to a method's reliability in real life, when people don't always use a method properly. For comparison, about 85 percent of sexually active women using no contraception would be expected to become pregnant in a year.

242

This chart is a summary; it is not intended to be used alone. All product labeling should be followed carefully, and a health-care professional should be consulted for some methods.

Male Condom

Estimated Effectiveness: 88% (a)

Some Risks (d): Irritation and allergic reactions (less likely with polyurethane)

Protection from Sexually Transmitted Diseases (STDs): Except for abstinence, latex condoms are the best protection against STDs, including herpes and AIDS.

Convenience: Applied immediately before intercourse; used only once and discarded.

Availability: Nonprescription

Female Condom

Estimated Effectiveness: 79%

Some Risks (d): Irritation and allergic reactions

Protection from Sexually Transmitted Diseases (STDs): May give some STD protection; not as effective as latex condom.

Convenience: Applied immediately before intercourse; used only once and discarded.

Availability: Nonprescription

Diaphragm with Spermicide

Estimated Effectiveness: 82%

Some Risks (d): Irritation and allergic reactions, urinary tract infection

Protection from Sexually Transmitted Diseases (STDs): Protects against cervical infection; spermicide may give some protection against chlamydia and gonorrhea; otherwise unknown.

Convenience: Inserted before intercourse and left in place at least six hours after; can be left in place for 24 hours, with additional spermicide for repeated intercourse.

Availability: Prescription

Cervical Cap with Spermicide

Estimated Effectiveness: 64-82% (b)

Some Risks (d): Irritation and allergic reactions, abnormal Pap test

Protection from Sexually Transmitted Diseases (STDs): Spermicide may give some protection against chlamydia and gonorrhea; otherwise unknown.

Convenience: May be difficult to insert; can remain in place for 48 hours without reapplying spermicide for repeated intercourse.

Availability: Prescription

Sponge with Spermicide (not currently marketed)

Estimated Effectiveness: 64-82% (b)

Some Risks (d): Irritation and allergic reactions, difficulty in removal

Protection from Sexually Transmitted Diseases (STDs): Spermicide may give some protection against chlamydia and gonorrhea; otherwise unknown.

Convenience: Inserted before intercourse and protects for 24 hours without additional spermicide; must be left in place for at least six hours after intercourse; must be removed within 30 hours of insertion; used only once and discarded.

Availability: Nonprescription; not currently marketed.

Spermicides Alone

Estimated Effectiveness: 79%

Some Risks (d): Irritation and allergic reactions

Protection from Sexually Transmitted Diseases (STDs): May give some protection against chlamydia and gonorrhea; otherwise unknown.

Convenience: Instructions vary; usually applied no more than one hour before intercourse and left in place at least six to eight hours after.

Availability: Nonprescription

Oral Contraceptives--combined pill

Estimated Effectiveness: Over 99% (c)

Some Risks (d): Dizziness; nausea; changes in menstruation, mood, and weight; rarely cardiovascular disease, including high blood pressure, blood clots, heart attack, and strokes

Protection from Sexually Transmitted Diseases (STDs): None, except some protection against pelvic inflammatory disease.

Convenience: Must be taken on daily schedule, regardless of frequency of intercourse.

Availability: Prescription

Oral Contraceptives--progestin-only minipill

Estimated Effectiveness: Over 99% (c)

Some Risks (d): Ectopic pregnancy, irregular bleeding, weight gain, breast tenderness

Protection from Sexually Transmitted Diseases (STDs): None, except some protection against pelvic inflammatory disease.

Convenience: Must be taken on daily schedule, regardless of frequency of intercourse.

Availability: Prescription

Injection (Depo-Provera)

Estimated Effectiveness: Over 99%

Some Risks (d): Irregular bleeding, weight gain, breast tenderness, headaches

Protection from Sexually Transmitted Diseases (STDs): None

Convenience: One injection every three months

Availability: Prescription

Implant (Norplant)

Estimated Effectiveness: Over 99%

Some Risks (d): Irregular bleeding, weight gain, breast tenderness, headaches, difficulty in removal

Protection from Sexually Transmitted Diseases (STDs): None

Convenience: Implanted by health-care provider--minor outpatient surgical procedure; effective for up to five years.

Availability: Prescription

IUD (Intrauterine Device)

Estimated Effectiveness: 98-99%

Some Risks (d): Cramps, bleeding, pelvic inflammatory disease, infertility, perforation of uterus

Protection from Sexually Transmitted Diseases (STDs): None

Convenience: After insertion by physician, can remain in place for up to one or 10 years, depending on type.

Availability: Prescription

Periodic Abstinence

Estimated Effectiveness: About 80% (variable, based on method)

Some Risks (d): None

Protection from Sexually Transmitted Diseases (STDs): None

Convenience: Requires frequent monitoring of body functions (for example, body temperature for one method).

Availability: Instructions from health-care provider

Surgical Sterilization--female or male

Estimated Effectiveness: Over 99%

Some Risks (d): Pain, bleeding, infection, other minor postsurgical complications

Protection from Sexually Transmitted Diseases (STDs): None

246

Convenience: One-time surgical procedure

Availability: Surgery

Footnotes

(a) Effectiveness rate for polyurethane condoms has not been established.

(b) Less effective for women who have had a baby because the birth process stretches the vagina and cervix, making it more difficult to achieve a proper fit.

(c) Based on perfect use, when the woman takes the pill every day as directed.

(d) Serious medical risks from contraceptives are rare.

References

Nordenberg, Tamar(1997) Protecting Against Unintended Pregnancy A Guide to Contraceptive Choices FDA Consumer magazine (April 1997)

Contraceptive Technology (16th edition, 1994)

Male Latex Condoms and Sexually Transmitted Diseases

In June 2000, the National Institutes of Health (NIH), in collaboration with the Centers for Disease Control and Prevention (CDC), the Food and Drug Administration (FDA), and the United States Agency for International Development (USAID), convened a workshop to evaluate the published evidence establishing the effectiveness of latex male condoms in preventing STDs, including HIV. A summary report from that workshop was completed in July 2001.

This fact sheet is based on the NIH workshop report and additional studies that were not reviewed in that report or were published subsequent to the workshop (see link for additional references). Most epidemiologic studies comparing rates of STD transmission between condom users and non-users focus on penile-vaginal intercourse.

Recommendations concerning the male latex condom and the prevention of sexually transmitted diseases (STDs), including human immunodeficiency virus (HIV), are based on information about how different STDs are transmitted, the physical properties of condoms, the anatomic coverage or protection that condoms provide, and epidemiologic studies of condom use and STD risk.

The surest way to avoid transmission of sexually transmitted diseases is to abstain from sexual intercourse, or to be in a long-term mutually monogamous relationship with a partner who has been tested and you know is uninfected.

For persons whose sexual behaviors place them at risk for STDs, correct and consistent use of the male latex condom can reduce the risk of STD transmission. However, no protective method is 100 percent effective, and condom use cannot guarantee absolute protection against any STD. Furthermore, condoms lubricated with spermicides are no more effective than other lubricated condoms in protecting against the transmission of HIV and other STDs. In order to achieve the protective effect of condoms, they must be used correctly and consistently. Incorrect use can lead to condom slippage or breakage, thus diminishing their protective effect. Inconsistent use, e.g., failure to use condoms with every act of intercourse, can lead to STD transmission because transmission can occur with a single act of intercourse. While condom use has been associated with a lower risk of cervical cancer, the use of condoms should not be a substitute for routine screening with Pap smears to detect and prevent cervical cancer.

Sexually transmitted diseases, including HIV

Latex condoms, when used consistently and correctly, are highly effective in preventing transmission of HIV, the virus that causes AIDS. In addition, correct and consistent use of latex condoms can reduce the risk of other sexually transmitted diseases (STDs), including discharge and genital ulcer diseases. While the effect of condoms in preventing human papillomavirus (HPV) infection is unknown, condom use has been associated with a lower rate of cervical cancer, an HPV-associated disease.

There are two primary ways that STDs can be transmitted. Human immunodeficiency virus (HIV), as well as gonorrhea, chlamydia, and trichomoniasis – the discharge diseases – are transmitted when infected semen or vaginal fluids contact mucosal surfaces (e.g., the male urethra, the vagina or cervix). In contrast, genital ulcer diseases – genital herpes, syphilis, and chancroid – and human papillomavirus are primarily transmitted through contact with infected skin or mucosal surfaces.

Laboratory studies have demonstrated that latex condoms provide an essentially impermeable barrier to particles the size of STD pathogens.

Theoretical basis for protection. Condoms can be expected to provide different levels of protection for various sexually transmitted diseases, depending on differences in how the diseases are transmitted. Because condoms block the discharge of semen or protect the male urethra against exposure to vaginal secretions, a greater level of protection is provided for the discharge diseases.

A lesser degree of protection is provided for the genital ulcer diseases or HPV because these infections may be transmitted by exposure to areas, e.g., infected skin or mucosal surfaces, that are not covered or protected by the condom.

Epidemiologic studies seek to measure the protective effect of condoms by comparing rates of STDs between condom users and nonusers in real-life settings. Developing such measures of condom effectiveness is challenging. Because these studies involve private behaviors that investigators cannot observe directly, it is difficult to determine accurately whether an individual is a condom user or whether condoms are used consistently and correctly. Likewise, it can be difficult to determine the level of exposure to STDs among study participants. These problems are often compounded in studies that employ a "retrospective" design, e.g., studies that measure behaviors and risks in the past.

As a result, observed measures of condom effectiveness may be inaccurate. Most epidemiologic studies of STDs, other than HIV, are characterized by these methodological limitations, and thus, the results across them vary widely--ranging from demonstrating no protection to demonstrating substantial protection associated with condom use. This inconclusiveness of epidemiologic data about condom effectiveness indicates that more research is needed--not that latex condoms do not work. For HIV infection, unlike other STDs, a number of carefully conducted studies, employing more rigorous methods and measures, have demonstrated that consistent condom use is a highly effective means of preventing HIV transmission.

Another type of epidemiologic study involves examination of STD rates in populations rather than individuals. Such studies have demonstrated that when condom use increases within population groups, rates of STDs decline in these groups. Other studies have examined the relationship between condom use and the complications of sexually transmitted infections. For example, condom use has been associated with a decreased risk of cervical cancer – an HPV associated disease.

Protection against HIV/AIDS

AIDS is, by far, the most deadly sexually transmitted disease, and considerably more scientific evidence exists regarding condom effectiveness for prevention of HIV infection than for other STDs. The body of research on the effectiveness of latex condoms in preventing sexual transmission of HIV is both comprehensive and conclusive. In fact, the ability of latex condoms to prevent transmission of HIV has been scientifically established in "real-life" studies of sexually active couples as well as in laboratory studies.

Laboratory studies have demonstrated that latex condoms provide an essentially impermeable barrier to particles the size of STD pathogens.

Theoretical basis for protection. Latex condoms cover the penis and provide an effective barrier to exposure to secretions such as semen and vaginal fluids, blocking the pathway of sexual transmission of HIV infection.

Epidemiologic studies that are conducted in real-life settings, where one partner is infected with HIV and the other partner is not, demonstrate conclusively that the consistent use of latex condoms provides a high degree of protection.

Discharge Diseases, Including Gonorrhea, Chlamydia, and Trichomoniasis

Gonorrhea, chlamydia, and trichomoniasis are termed discharge diseases because they are sexually transmitted by genital secretions, such as semen or vaginal fluids. HIV is also transmitted by genital secretions.

Laboratory studies have demonstrated that latex condoms provide an essentially impermeable barrier to particles the size of STD pathogens.

Theoretical basis for protection.

The physical properties of latex condoms protect against discharge diseases such as gonorrhea, chlamydia, and trichomoniasis, by providing a barrier to the genital secretions that transmit STD-causing organisms.

Epidemiologic studies that compare infection rates among condom users and nonusers provide evidence that latex condoms can protect against the transmission of chlamydia, gonorrhea and trichomoniasis. However, some other epidemiologic studies show little or no protection against these infections. Many of the available epidemiologic studies were not designed or conducted in ways that allow for accurate measurement of condom effectiveness against the discharge diseases. More research is needed to assess the degree of protection latex condoms provide for discharge diseases, other than HIV.

Genital Ulcer Diseases and Human Papillomavirus

Genital ulcer diseases and HPV infections can occur in both male and female genital areas that are covered or protected by a latex condom, as well as in areas that are not covered. Correct and consistent use of latex condoms can reduce the risk of genital herpes, syphilis, and chancroid only when the infected area or site of potential exposure is protected. While the effect of condoms in preventing human papillomavirus infection is unknown, condom use has been associated with a lower rate of cervical cancer, an HPV-associated disease.

Genital ulcer diseases include genital herpes, syphilis, and chancroid. These diseases are transmitted primarily through "skin-to-skin" contact from sores/ulcers or infected skin that looks normal. HPV infections are transmitted through contact with infected genital skin or mucosal surfaces/fluids. Genital ulcer diseases and HPV infection can occur in male or female genital areas that are, or are not, covered (protected by the condom).

Laboratory studies have demonstrated that latex condoms provide an essentially impermeable barrier to particles the size of STD pathogens.

Theoretical basis for protection. Protection against genital ulcer diseases and HPV depends on the site of the sore/ulcer or infection. Latex condoms can only protect against transmission when the ulcers or infections are in genital areas that are covered or protected by the condom. Thus, consistent and correct use of latex condoms would be expected to protect against transmission of genital ulcer diseases and HPV in some, but not all, instances.

Epidemiologic studies that compare infection rates among condom users and nonusers provide evidence that latex condoms can protect against the transmission of syphilis and genital herpes. However, some other epidemiologic studies show little or no protection. Many of the available epidemiologic studies were not designed or conducted in ways that allow for accurate measurement of condom effectiveness against the genital ulcer diseases. No conclusive studies have specifically addressed the transmission of chancroid and condom use, although several studies have documented a reduced risk of genital ulcers in settings where chancroid is a leading cause of genital ulcers. More research is needed to assess the degree of protection latex condoms provide for the genital ulcer diseases.

While some epidemiologic studies have demonstrated lower rates of HPV infection among condom users, most have not. It is particularly difficult to study the relationship between condom use and HPV infection because HPV infection is often intermittently detectable and because it is difficult to assess the frequency of either existing or new infections. Many of the available epidemiologic studies were not designed or conducted in ways that allow for accurate measurement of condom effectiveness against HPV infection.

A number of studies, however, do show an association between condom use and a reduced risk of HPV-associated diseases, including genital warts, cervical dysplasia and cervical cancer. The reason for lower rates of cervical cancer among condom users observed in some studies is unknown. HPV infection is believed to be required, but not by itself sufficient, for cervical cancer to occur. Co-infections with other STDs may be a factor in increasing the likelihood that HPV infection will lead to cervical cancer. More research is needed to assess the degree of protection latex condoms provide for both HPV infection and HPV-associated disease, such as cervical cancer.

References

Workshop Summary: July 20, 2001 Scientific Evidence on Condom Effectiveness for Sexually Transmitted Disease (STD) Prevention, June 12-13, 2000 National Institute of Allergy and Infectious Diseases, National Institutes of Health, Department of Health and Human Services. (http://www.niaid.nih.gov/dmid/stds/condomreport.pdf).

Important Parasites

As medical science has become more precise in diagnosing different infectious diseases, the list of known sexually transmitted diseases (STDs) has grown. The earlier sections dealt with the major STDs that are common in the United States: chlamydial infections; gonorrhea; pelvic inflammatory disease (PID); trichomoniasis and other vaginal infections; syphilis; genital herpes; genital warts; AIDS; and hepatitis.

This chapter provides information on some of the parasites that can be transmitted sexually: pubic "crab" lice and scabies

.Pubic Lice Infestation

What are pubic lice?

Also called "crabs," pubic lice are parasitic insects found in the genital area of humans. Infection is common and found worldwide.

How did I get pubic lice?

Pubic lice are usually spread through sexual contact. Rarely, infestation can be spread through contact with an infested person's bed linens, towels, or clothes. A common misunderstanding is that infestation can be spread by sitting on a toilet seat. This isn't likely, since lice cannot live long away from a warm human body. Also, lice do not have feet designed to walk or hold onto smooth surfaces such as toilet seats.

Infection in a young child or teenager may indicate sexual activity or sexual abuse.

Where are pubic lice found?

Pubic lice are generally found in the genital area on pubic hair; but may occasionally be found on other coarse body hair, such as hair on the legs, armpits, mustache, beard, eyebrows, or eyelashes. Infestations of young children are usually on the eyebrows or eyelashes. Lice found on the head are not pubic lice; they are head lice.

Animals do not get or spread pubic lice.

What are the signs and symptoms of pubic lice?

Signs and symptoms of pubic lice include

- Itching in the genital area
- Visible nits (lice eggs) or crawling lice

What do pubic lice look like?

There are three stages in the life of a pubic louse: the nit, the nymph, and the adult.

Nit: Nits are pubic lice eggs. They are hard to see and are found firmly attached to the hair shaft.

They are about the size of the mark at the end of this arrow → '. They are oval and usually yellow to white. Nits take about 1 week to hatch.

Nymph: The nit hatches into a baby louse called a nymph. It looks like an adult pubic louse, but it is smaller. Nymphs mature into adults about 7 days after hatching. To live, the nymph must feed on blood.

Adult: The adult pubic louse is about the size of this circle → Oand resembles a miniature crab when viewed through a strong magnifying glass. Pubic lice have six legs, but their two front legs are very large and look like the pincher claws of a crab; this is how they got the nickname "crabs." Pubic lice are tan to grayish-white in color. Females lay nits and are usually larger than males. To live, adult lice must feed on blood. If the louse falls off a person, it dies within 1-2 days.

How is a pubic lice infestation diagnosed?

A lice infestation is diagnosed by looking closely through pubic hair for nits, nymphs, or adults. It may be difficult to find nymph or adult; here are usually few of them and they can move quickly away from light. If crawling lice are not seen, finding nits confirms that a person is infested and should be treated. If you are unsure about infestation or if treatment is not successful, see a health care provider for a diagnosis.

How is a pubic lice infestation treated?

A lice-killing shampoo (also called a pediculicide) made of 1% permethrin or pyrethrin is recommended to treat pubic lice. These products are available without a prescription at your local drug store. Medication is generally very effective; apply the medication exactly as directed on the bottle. A prescription medication, called Lindane (1%) is available through your health care provider. Lindane is not recommended for pregnant or nursing women, or for children less than 2 years old.

Malathion* lotion 0.5% (Ovide*) is another prescription medication that is effective against pubic lice.

How to treat pubic lice infestations: (Note: see section below for treatment of eyelashes or eyebrows. The lice medications described in this section should not be used near the eyes.)

- Wash the infested area; towel dry.
- Thoroughly saturate hair with lice medication. If using permethrin or pyrethrins, leave medication on for 10 minutes; if using Lindane, only leave on for 4 minutes. Thoroughly rinse off medication with water. Dry off with a clean towel.
- Following treatment, most nits will still be attached to hair shafts. Nits may be removed with fingernails.
- Put on clean underwear and clothing after treatment.
- To kill any lice or nits (attached to hairs) that may be left on clothing or bedding, machine-wash those washable items that the infested person used during the 2-3 days before treatment. Use the hot water cycle (130°F). Use the hot dryer cycle for at least 20 minutes.
- Dry-clean clothing that is not washable.
- Inform any sexual partners that they are at risk for infestation.
- Do not have sex until treatment is complete.

- Do not have sex with infected partners until partners have been treated and infestation has been cured.

- Repeat treatment in 7-10 days if lice are still found.

To treat nits and lice found on eyebrows or eyelashes:

- If only a few nits are found, it may be possible to remove live lice and nits with your fingernails or a nit comb.

- If additional treatment is needed for pubic lice nits found on the eyelashes, applying an ophthalmic-grade petrolatum ointment (only available by prescription) to the eyelids twice a day for 10 days is effective. Vaseline* is a kind of petrolatum, but is likely to irritate the eyes if applied.

Use of trade names is for identification purposes only and does not imply endorsement by the Public Health Service or by the U.S. Department of Health and Human Services.

Head Lice Infestation
Pediculosis

What are head lice?

Also called *Pediculus humanus capitis* (peh-DICK-you-lus HUE-man-us CAP-ih-TUS), head lice are parasitic insects found on the heads of people. Having head lice is very common. However, there are no reliable data on how many people get head lice in the United States each year.

Who is at risk for getting head lice?

Anyone who comes in close contact (especially head-to-head contact) with someone who already has head lice is at greatest risk. Occasionally, head lice may be acquired from contact with clothing (such as hats, scarves, coats) or other personal items (such as brushes or towels) that belong to an infested person. Preschool and elementary-age children, 3-11, and their families are infested most often. Girls get head lice more often than boys, women more than men. In the United States, African-Americans rarely get head lice. Personal hygiene or cleanliness in the home or school has nothing to do with getting head lice.

What do head lice look like?

There are three forms of lice: the egg (also called a nit), the nymph, and the adult.

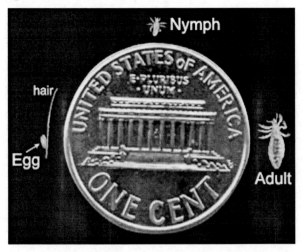

Actual size of the three lice forms compared to a penny *(Photo credit: CDC)*

Egg/Nit: Nits are head lice eggs. They are very small, about the size of a knot in thread, hard to see, and are often confused for dandruff or hair spray droplets. Nits are laid by the adult female at the base of the hair shaft nearest the scalp. They are firmly attached to the hair shaft. They are oval and usually yellow to white. Nits take about 1 week to hatch. Eggs that are likely to hatch are usually located within 1/4 inch of the scalp.

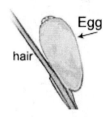

Illustration of egg on a hair shaft
(Image credit: CDC)

Nymph: The nit hatches into a baby louse called a nymph. It looks like an adult head louse, but is smaller. Nymphs mature into adults about 7 days after hatching. To live, the nymph must feed on blood.

Nymph form
(Photo credit: CDC)

Adult: The adult louse is about the size of a sesame seed, has six legs, and is tan to greyish-white. In persons with dark hair, the adult louse will look darker. Females, which are usually larger than the males, lay eggs. Adult lice can live up to 30 days on a person's head. To live, adult lice need to feed on blood. If the louse falls off a person, it dies within 2 days.

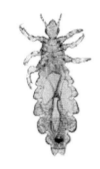

Adult louse
(Image credit: CDC)

Where are head lice most commonly found?

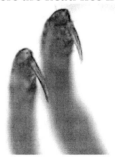

Adult louse claws
(Photo credit: CDC)

They are most commonly found on the scalp, behind the ears and near the neckline at the back of the neck. Head lice hold on to hair with hook-like claws found at the end of each of their six legs. Head lice are rarely found on the body, eyelashes, or eyebrows.

260

What are the signs and symptoms of head lice infestation?

- Tickling feeling of something moving in the hair.

- Itching, caused by an allergic reaction to the bites.

- Irritability.

- Sores on the head caused by scratching. These sores can sometimes become infected.

How did my child get head lice?

Contact with an already infested person is the most common way to get head lice. Head-to-head contact is common during play at school and at home (sports activities, on a playground, slumber parties, at camp).

Less commonly,

- Wearing clothing, such as hats, scarves, coats, sports uniforms, or hair ribbons, recently worn by an infested person.

- Using infested combs, brushes, or towels.

- Lying on a bed, couch, pillow, carpet, or stuffed animal that has recently been in contact with an infested person.

How is head lice infestation diagnosed?

An infestation is diagnosed by looking closely through the hair and scalp for nits, nymphs, or adults. Finding a nymph or adult may be difficult; there are usually few of them and they can move quickly from searching fingers.

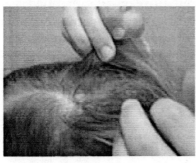

If crawling lice are not seen, finding nits within a 1/4 inch of the scalp confirms that a person is infested and should be treated. If you only find nits more than 1/4 inch from the scalp (and don't see a nymph or adult louse), the

(Photo Credit: CDC)

infestation is probably an old one and does not need to be treated. If you are not sure if a person has head lice, the diagnosis should be made by your health care provider, school nurse, or a professional from the local health department or agricultural extension service.

Treating Head Lice Infestation

How can I treat a head lice infestation?

The most important step in treating a head lice infestation is to treat the person and other family members with head lice with medication to kill the lice. Wash clothing and bedding worn or used by the infested person in the 2-day period just before treatment is started.

Treat the infested person: Requires using an over-the-counter (OTC) or prescription medication. Follow these treatment steps:

- Before applying treatment, remove all clothing from the waist up.

- Apply lice medicine, also called pediculicide (peh-DICK-you-luh-side), according to label instructions. If your child has extra long hair (longer than shoulder length), you may need to use a second bottle. Pay special attention to instructions on the bottle regarding how long the medication should be left on and whether rinsing the hair is recommended after treatment.

WARNING: Do not use a creme rinse or combination shampoo/conditioner before using lice medicine. Do not re-wash hair for 1-2 days after treatment.

- Have the infested person put on clean clothing after treatment.

- If a few live lice are still found 8-12 hours after treatment, but are moving more slowly than before, do not retreat. Comb dead and remaining live lice out of the hair. The medicine may take longer to kill lice.

- If, after 8-12 hours of treatment, no dead lice are found and lice seem as active as before, the medicine may not be working. See your health care provider for a different medication; follow treatment directions.

- Nit (head lice egg) combs, often found in lice medicine packages, should be used to comb nits and lice from the hair shaft. Many flea combs made for cats and dogs are also effective.

- After treatment, check hair and comb with a nit comb to remove nits and lice every 2-3 days. Continue to check for 2-3 weeks until you are sure all lice and nits are gone.

- If using OTC pediculicides, retreat in 7-10 days. If using the prescription drug malathion, retreat in 7-10 days ONLY if crawling bugs are found.

Treat the household: Head lice do not survive long if they fall off a person and cannot feed. You don't need to spend a lot of time or money on housecleaning activities. Follow these steps to help avoid re-infestation by lice that have recently fallen off the hair or crawled onto clothing or furniture.

- To kill lice and nits, machine wash all washable clothing and bed linens that the infested person wore or used during the 2 days before treatment. Use the hot water (130°F) cycle. Dry laundry using high heat for at least 20 minutes.

- Dry clean clothing that is not washable, (coats, hats, scarves, etc.).

OR

- Store all clothing, stuffed animals, comforters, etc., that cannot be washed or dry cleaned into a plastic bag; seal for 2 weeks.

- Soak combs and brushes for 1 hour in rubbing alcohol, Lysol*, or wash with soap and hot (130°F) water.

- Vacuum the floor and furniture. The risk of getting re-infested from a louse that has fallen onto a carpet or sofa is very small. Don't spend a lot of time on this. Just vacuum the places where the infested person usually sits or lays. Do not use fumigant sprays; they can be toxic if inhaled or absorbed through the skin.

Prevent Reinfestation: Lice are most commonly spread directly by head-to-head contact and much less frequently by lice that have crawled onto clothing or belongings. As a short-term measure to control a head lice outbreak in a community, school, or camp, you can teach children to avoid playtime and other activities that are likely to spread lice.

- Avoid head-to-head contact common during play at school and at home (sports activities, on a playground, slumber parties, at camp).

- Do not share clothing, such as hats, scarves, coats, sports uniforms, or hair ribbons.

- Do not share infested combs, brushes, or towels.

- Do not lie on beds, couches, pillows, carpets, or stuffed animals that have recently been in contact with an infested person.

My child has head lice. I don't. Should I treat myself to prevent being infested?

No, although anyone living with an infested person can get head lice. Check household contacts for lice and nits every 2-3 days. Treat only if crawling lice or nits (eggs) within a 1/4 inch of the scalp are found.

I have heard that head lice medications don't work, or that head lice are resistant to medication. Is this true?
Like germs that are resistant to antibiotics, some lice also develop resistance to the medicine used to kill them. Resistance tends to be scattered. It may be present in one neighborhood, but not another. However, there are many reasons why medications may seem not to work.

Misdiagnosis of a head lice infestation. A diagnosis can be made if a person has crawling bugs on the head or many lice eggs within 1/4 inch (about the width of your little finger) of the scalp. Nits found on the hair shaft further than 1/4 inch from the scalp have already hatched. Treatment is not recommended for people who only have nits further than 1/4 inch away from the scalp.

Not following treatment instructions fully. Common problems include:

- making the hair too wet with water before applying a pediculicide — this dilutes the pediculicide

- using a creme rinse or conditioner shampoo before applying a pediculicide — this interferes with the medication

- failure to leave the pediculicide on long enough — follow drug label instructions

- re-shampooing the hair again immediately after applying the pediculicide — don't rewash hair for 1-2 days after treatment

- inadequate amount of medication — extra long hair may require two bottles of pediculide to fully wet the hair

- not combing. Using medication alone may not be enough to cure a head lice infestation. Combing the hair to remove lice and eggs has been shown to help.

Medication not working at all (resistance). If head lice medication does not kill any crawling bugs within 24 hours, then resistance is likely. If the medication kills some of the bugs or the bugs are twitching 24 hours after treatment then resistance to medication is probably not occurring.

Medication kills crawling bugs, but is not able to penetrate the eggs. It is very difficult for head lice medication to penetrate the nit shell. Medication may effectively kill crawling bugs, but may not treat the nits. This is why follow-up treatment is recommended.

New infection. You can get infested more than once with head lice. Children often get re-infested from a playmate. If your child is infested, discuss it with parents of the children your child plays with. Treating all infested children at the same time will help prevent reinfestation.

Should my pets be treated for head lice?

No. Head lice do not live on pets.

My child is under 2 years old and has been diagnosed with head lice. Can I treat him or her with prescription or OTC drugs?

For children under 2 years old, remove crawling bugs and nits using a nit comb. If this does not work, ask your child's health care provider for treatment recommendations. The safety of head lice medications has not been tested in children 2 years of age and under.

What OTC medications are available to treat head lice?

Many head lice medications are available at your local drug store. Each OTC product contains one of the following active ingredients.

- **Pyrethrins** (pie-WREATH-rins) — often combined with piperonyl butoxide (pie-PER-a-nil beu-TOX-side):
- Brand name products include A-200*, Pronto*, R&C*, Rid*, Triple X*.

Pyrethrins are natural extracts from the chrysanthemum flower. Though safe and effective, pyrethrins only kill crawling lice, not unhatched nits. A second treatment is recommended in 7-10 days to kill any newly hatched lice. Treatment failures are common.

- **Permethrin** (per-meth-rin):Brand name product: Nix*.

Permethrins are similar to natural pyrethrins. Permethrins are safe and effective and may continue to kill newly hatched lice for several days after treatment. A second treatment may be necessary in 7-10 days to kill any newly hatched lice that may have hatched after residual medication from the first treatment was no longer active. Treatment failures are common.

What are the prescription drugs used to treat head lice?

- **Malathion** (Ovide*): When used as directed, malathion is effective in treating lice. Some medication remains on the hair and can kill newly hatched lice for seven days after treatment. Malathion is intended for use on people 6 years of age and older. Few side-effects have been reported. Malathion may sting if applied to open sores caused by scratching. The medication is flammable.

- **Lindane** (Kwell*): When used as directed, the drug is probably safe. Overuse, misuse, or accidentally swallowing Lindane can be toxic to the brain and other parts of the nervous system. For those reasons Lindane is generally used only if other medications have failed. Lindane should not be used if excessive scratching has caused open sores on the head. It should be used with caution in persons who weigh less than 110 pounds.

Which head lice medicine is best for me?

If you aren't sure, ask your pharmacist or health care provider. When using the medicine, always follow the instructions provided.

When treating head lice

- Do not use extra amounts of the lice medication unless instructed. These drugs are insecticides and can be dangerous when misused or overused.

- Do not treat the infested person more than 3 times with the same medication if it does not seem to work. See your health care provider for alternative medication.

- Do not mix head lice drugs.

Should household sprays be used to kill adult lice?

No. Spraying the house is NOT recommended. Fumigants and room sprays can be toxic if inhaled or absorbed through the skin.

Should I have a pest control company spray my house?

No. Vacuuming floors and furniture is enough to treat the household.

Use of trade names is for identification purposes only and does not imply endorsement by the Public Health Service or by the U.S. Department of Health and Human Services

Scabies
(SKAY-bees)

What is scabies?

Scabies is an infestation of the skin with the microscopic mite Sarcoptes scabei. Infestation is common, found worldwide, and affects people of all races and social classes. Scabies spreads rapidly under crowded conditions where there is frequent skin-to-skin contact between people, such as in hospitals, institutions, child-care facilities, and nursing homes.

What are the signs and symptoms of scabies infestation?

- Pimple-like irritations, burrows or rash of the skin, especially the webbing between the fingers; the skin folds on the wrist, elbow, or knee; the penis, the breast, or shoulder blades.

- Intense itching, especially at night and over most of the body.

- Sores on the body caused by scratching. These sores can sometimes become infected with bacteria.

How did I get scabies?

By direct, prolonged, skin-to-skin contact with a person already infested with scabies. Contact must be prolonged (a quick handshake or hug will usually not spread infestation). Infestation is easily spread to sexual partners and household members. Infestation may also occur by sharing clothing, towels, and bedding.

Who is at risk for severe infestation?

People with weakened immune systems and the elderly are at risk for a more severe form of scabies, called Norwegian or crusted scabies.

How long will mites live?

Once away from the human body, mites do not survive more than 48-72 hours. When living on a person, an adult female mite can live up to a month.

Did my pet spread scabies to me?

No. Pets become infested with a different kind of scabies mite. If your pet is infested with scabies, (also called mange) and they have close contact with you, the mite can get under your skin and cause itching and skin irritation. However, the mite dies in a couple of days and does not reproduce. The mites may cause you to itch for several days, but you do not need to be treated with special medication to kill the mites. Until your pet is successfully treated, mites can continue to burrow into your skin and cause you to have symptoms.

How soon after infestation will symptoms begin?

For a person who has never been infested with scabies, symptoms may take 4-6 weeks to begin. For a person who has had scabies, symptoms appear within several days. You do not become immune to an infestation.

How is scabies infestation diagnosed?

Diagnosis is most commonly made by looking at the burrows or rash. A skin scraping may be taken to look for mites, eggs, or mite fecal matter to confirm the diagnosis. If a skin scraping or biopsy is taken and returns negative, it is possible that you may still be infested. Typically, there are fewer than 10 mites on the entire body of an infested person; this makes it easy for an infestation to be missed.

Can scabies be treated?

Yes. Several lotions are available to treat scabies. Always follow the directions provided by your physician or the directions on the package insert. Apply lotion to a clean body from the neck down to the toes and left overnight (8 hours). After 8 hours, take a bath or shower to wash off the lotion. Put on clean clothes. All clothes, bedding, and towels used by the infested person 2 days before treatment should be washed in hot water; dry in a hot dryer. A second treatment of the body with the same lotion may be necessary 7-10 days later. Pregnant women and children are often treated with milder scabies medications.

Who should be treated for scabies?

Anyone who is diagnosed with scabies, as well as his or her sexual partners and persons who have close, prolonged contact to the infested person should also be treated. If your health care provider has instructed family members to be treated, everyone should receive treatment at the same time to prevent reinfestation.

How soon after treatment will I feel better?

Itching may continue for 2-3 weeks, and does not mean that you are still infested. Your health care provider my prescribe additional medication to relieve itching if it is severe. No new burrows or rashes should appear 24-48 hours after effective treatment.

Causal Agent:

Sarcoptes scabei, human itch or mange mites, are in the arthropod class Arachnida, subclass Acari, family Sarcoptidae. The mites burrow into the skin but never below the stratum corneum. The burrows appear as raised serpentine lines up to several centimeters long. Other races of scabies may cause infestations in other mammals such as domestic cats, dogs, pigs, and horses. It should be noted that races of mites found on other animals may establish infestations in humans. They may cause temporary itching due to dermatitis but they do not multiply on the human host.

Life Cycle:

Sarcoptes scabei undergoes four stages in its life cycle; egg, larva, nymph and adult. Females deposit eggs at 2 to 3 day intervals as they burrow through the skin ❶. Eggs are oval and 0.1 to 0.15 mm in length ❷ and incubation time is 3 to 8 days. After the eggs hatch, the larvae migrate to the skin surface and burrow into the intact stratum corneum to construct almost invisible, short burrows called molting pouches. The larval stage, which emerges from the eggs, has only 3 pairs of legs ❸, and this form lasts 2 to 3 days. After larvae molt, the resulting nymphs have 4 pairs of legs ❹. This form molts into slightly larger nymphs before molting into adults. Larvae and nymphs may often be found in molting pouches or in hair follicles and look similar to adults, only smaller.

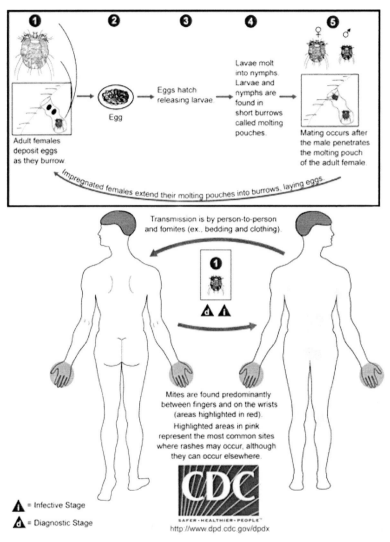

① Adult females deposit eggs as they burrow.

② Egg

Eggs hatch releasing larvae.

③ Lavae molt into nymphs. Larvae and nymphs are found in short burrows called molting pouches.

④ Mating occurs after the male penetrates the molting pouch of the adult female.

⑤

Impregnated females extend their molting pouches into burrows, laying eggs.

Transmission is by person-to-person and fomites (ex., bedding and clothing).

①

Mites are found predominantly between fingers and on the wrists (areas highlighted in red). Highlighted areas in pink represent the most common sites where rashes may occur, although they can occur elsewhere.

CDC

SAFER · HEALTHIER · PEOPLE™

http://www.dpd.cdc.gov/dpdx

△ = Infective Stage
△d = Diagnostic Stage

Adults are round, sac-like eyeless mites. Females are 0.3 to 0.4 mm long and 0.25 to 0.35 mm wide, and males are slightly more than half that size. Mating occurs after the nomadic male penetrates the molting pouch of the adult female ⑤. Impregnated females extend their molting pouches into the characteristic serpen-

272

tine burrows, laying eggs in the process. The impregnated females burrow into the skin and spend the remaining 2 months of their lives in tunnels under the surface of the skin. Males are rarely seen. They make a temporary gallery in the skin before mating.

Transmission occurs by the transfer of ovigerous females during personal contact. Mode of transmission is primarily person to person contact, but transmission may also occur via fomites (e.g., bedding or clothing). Mites are found predominantly between the fingers and on the wrists. The mites hold onto the skin using suckers attached to the two most anterior pairs of legs.

Geographic Distribution:
Scabies mites are distributed worldwide, affecting all races and socioeconomic classes in all climates.

Clinical Features:
When a person is infested with scabies mites for the first time, there is usually little evidence of infestation for the first month (range 2 to 6 weeks).

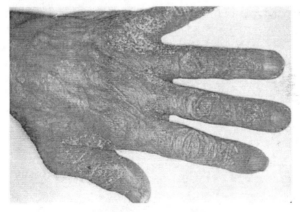

Scabies lesions are caused by Sarcoptes scabei burrowing under the skin. A typical location is on the hands, particularly the webbing between the fingers, as shown in this image. (CDC)

After this time and in subsequent infestations, people usually become sensitized to mites and symptoms generally occur within 1 to 4 days. Mites burrowing under the skin cause a rash, which is most frequently found on the hands, particularly the webbing between the fingers; the folds of the wrist, elbow or knee; the penis; the breast; or the shoulder blades.

Burrows and mites may be few in number and difficult to find in some cases. A papular "scabies rash" may be seen in skin areas where female mites are absent, usually on the buttocks, scapular region and abdomen; this may be a result of sensitization from a previous infection. Most commonly there is severe itching, especially at night and frequently over much of the body, including areas where mites are undetectable. A more severe form of scabies that is more common among immunocompromised persons is called Norwegian scabies, characterized by vesicles and formation of thick crusts over the skin, accompanied by abundant mites but only slight itching. Complications due to infestation are usually caused by secondary bacterial infections from scratching.

Laboratory Diagnosis:

Most diagnoses of scabies infestation are made based upon the appearance and distribution of the rash and the presence of burrows. Whenever possible scabies should be confirmed by isolating the mites, ova or feces in a skin scraping. Scrapings should be made at the burrows, especially on the hands between the fingers and the folds of the wrist. Alternatively, mites can be extracted from a burrow by gently pricking open the burrow with a needle and working it toward the end where the mite is living.

Diagnostic findings

Microscopy

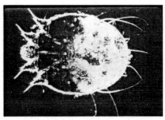

A: Sarcoptes scabei mite. Females are 0.3 to 0.4 mm long and 0.25 to 0.35 mm wide. Males are slightly more than half that size. The images in this section are from the CDC Division of Parasitic Diseases

Cross Section of Skin

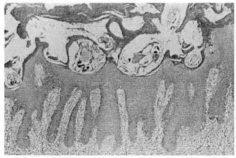

Cross sectional view of the burrows created in the epithelium by Sarcoptes scabei.

Treatment:

Several lotions are available to treat scabies. The treatment of choice is the topical use of permethrin (5%). Crotamiton and ivermectin* are alternative drugs. Ivermectin* is taken orally and is effective for treating crusted scabies in immunocompromised persons. If a topical preparation is used, a second treatment with the same product may be necessary 7-10 days later. All clothes, bedding, and towels used by the infested person during the 2 days before treatment should be washed in hot water, and dried in a hot dryer.

Statistics and STDs

The Mathematics of Risky Relationships

Robert J. Banis, PhD

A singular distinguishing characteristic of infections considered "sexually transmitted" is that the organisms are not very viable outside a human host. Sexually transmitted diseases (STDs) are not necessarily transmitted sexually, but are generally classified as STDs because intimate contact is the most likely route of transmission. In some cases, infections can be passed through bodily fluids that have been stored for some time. Such is the case for transmission of **Human Immunodeficiency Virus** (HIV), Cytomegalovirus (CMV) and Hepatitis in blood products. Neisseria gonorrhoeae, and Treponema pallidum, the bacteria that cause gonorrhea and syphilis, respectively, are more labile outside the body and don't survive in blood stored at refrigerator temperatures for more than a few days.

A "sexually transmitted infection" (STI) is unlikely to be contracted except through a relationship that involves exchange of bodily fluids, and the only way to be exposed is through a relationship that involves more than two people.

Thus, a sexually transmitted infection cannot survive in a monogamous or celibate culture, as it could not propagate and would eventually die out.

Your probability of being infected depends on:

- **Prevalence**—Probability your partner is infected
- **Infectivity**—Probability of transmission on a single exposure
- **Number of exposures**

Prevalence depends on the reproductive rate of the infection, defined as the number of people, on average, infected by an infected person over his lifetime. If the rate is one, the prevalence will be static, if less than one, it will eventually die out. Prevalence can only increase if the transmission rate is greater than the death rate.

The reproductive rate, sometimes called "infectee number" of an infected party is affected by:
- **Duration** of infectiousness
- **Probability of transmission** on a single exposure
- **Frequency** or number of exposure events
- **Rate of acquisition of new partners**

Prevalence & Approximate Transmission Characteristics				
Infection	Prevalence (USA) Per 100,000	Male to Female Pi	Female to Male Pi	Estimated Condom Protection
HIV-1	380	0.001-0.002	0.0005	Up to 90%
Gonorrhea	113.5	0.4	0.25	Variable up to 50%
Herpes (HSV-2)	25,000	0.001	0.001	Variable 30-50%
Syphilis	11.5	0.30	0.30	60-70%

Prevalence

Figures in the table refer to Centers for Disease Control (CDC) estimates of average incidence per 100,000 population.

This obviously varies substantially in different ethnic and cultural subgroups, such as men who have sex with men (MSM), Sexworkers, illegal injectable drug users (IDU), and in different age groups. Diseases that are non-lethal or are treatable but not curable, such as Herpes Simplex Virus (HSV), CMV, and Human Papilloma Virus (HPV) would be expected to be more prevalent in older age groups simply because they accumulate as cohorts age.

Diseases that are curable and with sufficient symptoms to be evident such as syphilis, gonorrhea, chlamydia and trichomoniasis would probably be more prevalent in younger age groups because younger people are more likely to be sexually active with multiple partners, but cures would be sought. Few STDs induce immunity after infection, so reinfection is relevant after one has been "cured." However, as subjects get older, they are more likely to be involved in relationships that reduce the turnover of partners, and so those who are cured are less likely to be reinfected.

Even though gonorrhea is asymptomatic in most females (or at least not noticed), as infected females mature and become involved in one-partner relationships the gonorrhea would become evident when it is inevitably transmitted to the male partner, who is more likely to display symptoms.

Detection of Asymptomatic Gonorrhea in Females when their Male Partners Become Infected and Show Symptoms

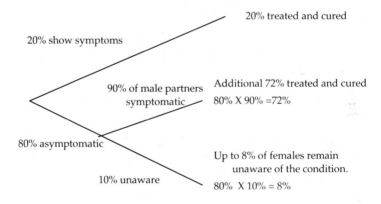

20% treated and cured

20% show symptoms

90% of male partners symptomatic

Additional 72% treated and cured
80% X 90% =72%

80% asymptomatic

10% unaware

Up to 8% of females remain unaware of the condition.
80% X 10% = 8%

Females are more likely to be asymptomatic but the infection is likely to be detected and treated after transmission to the male partner. For example, if 80% of females and 10% of males show symptoms of gonorrhea, and the probability of transmission to a monogamous male partner is close to 100% over some period of time, then 90% of the asymptomatic females would discover the problem when their partners exhibit the disease, and presumably, both partners would then be treated and cured.

HIV/AIDS and Hepatitis C are more likely to shorten lives, and so are more frequent in younger subjects who don't live to be infected older adults.

Prevalence is also affected by ease of transmission and by factors that affect detectability. Stealth infections are less likely to invoke protective behavior.

Thus, HSV, although it is not remarkably more infectious than HIV, has a much higher prevalence, possibly in part attributable to the fact that up to 90% of carriers are unaware of the infection.

CMV is more easily transmitted without intimate contact, is usually only evident in patients with immunological deficiencies and is estimated to have a prevalence of about 50-85% in adults by age 40.

See the earlier chapters on **Trends** for detailed information on prevalence of infections in various subgroups.

Treatment Effects on Duration of infectiousness

The length of time a subject is infectious is most obviously affected by curability and mortality.

In addition, virulence often varies as a function of stage of the infection.

Studies on HIV infectivity by Pinkerton and Abramson (1996) indicated infectivity was highest at two stages—in the first few months after infection, before antibodies were produced, and at the end of the asymptomatic period, when the body's defenses are overwhelmed. Thus infectivity is highest in the earliest stages, before seroconversion and before the infection is detectable. After that, symptoms of opportunistic infections become evident, and the subject, as well as potential sex partners, become aware of the infection. At this point, there may be behavioral changes that reduce transmission to future partners.

Unfortunately, a culture has been noted among MSM, that, since HIV/AIDS is treatable (with public aid) and since, barring a lifestyle change, infection is "inevitable," it is better to deliberately follow high-risk exposure patterns, catch the disease, and "get it over with." Under these circumstances, awareness of infection may have little effect on behavioral change.

Treatment of HIV/AIDS has been suggested to potentially give a perverse result, in which the eventual death rates in a population are increased by treating patients and thus extending their infective lifetimes (Anderson, et al., 2000).

On the other hand, HIV chemotherapy reduces the viral load and thus infectivity (Levin, et al, 2000).

Some diseases, such as syphilis, lapse into a dormant stage after the initial virulent infection, so after about a year, syphilis is no longer very infectious, but can progress into tertiary syphilis which can affect a variety of organs, including the brain (neuro-syphilis). Since the organism can't be cultured in vitro for direct observation, in the latent phase, diagnosis depends on VDRL and treponemal antibody titers which may suffer from a false negative interpretation.

The cure of syphilis by a single injection of natural Penicillin G wasn't discovered until 1941. Prior to that discovery, syphilis was not curable and the reported incidence in the United States in 1941 was 368 cases per 100,000 population. Use of penicillin drastically reduced the rate to 11.5 cases per 100,000 in 2004.

Probability of infection from a single incident

For easily transmitted STDs such as gonorrhea and syphilis, the probability of infection from a single incident has been estimated from studies of high risk high partner turnover situations such as sexworkers.

The risk for acquiring an infection from a single exposure to a person known to be infected has been estimated by for HIV and HSV-2 by studies with monogamous discordant couples who practice unprotected sex. Discordant couples are sex partners in a relationship where one of them has the infection and the other does not. Infectivity over a period of time involving a number of exposures is measured by the proportion of such couples in the study that experience conversion of the uninfected partner. The probability of infection on one exposure is back-calculated from this observation over time. This estimate of infectivity may be low compared to other populations. Factors affecting the probability of transmission include the presence of active HSV lesions, the type of sexual intercourse (i.e., oral, vaginal, or anal); any lesions or trauma (including bleeding); viral load in the bodily fluid transmitted; and presence of an STD or genital lesions in either party.

Thus, estimations of infectivity should be considered approximate in the context of the specific conditions of the cases observed in the study. Nevertheless, it's instructive to review the structure of the probability determinations to better understand the theory of infectivity over time in different types of relationships.

The estimate for infectivity, or probability of infection from a single incident, is back-calculated from the probability of infection over a period of time, taking into account the number of exposures over that period of time. This is not just a matter of dividing the overall probability by the number of incidents. Rather, it is the joint probability of transmission at least once in a long chain of events.

The best way to illustrate this is with a tree where there is a branch point with each exposure in which the exposure results either in transmission or not. If the probability of infection on a single contact is P_i, then the probability that the infection is not transmitted is $(1-P_i)$. Since these are sequential events and there are two branches at every event, the eventual number of paths, or possible permutations, is two to the power of the number of incidents. If the couple has 100 sexual contacts per year, one year would be represented by 2^{100} paths.

Joint probabilities for each of the paths would be the product of the individual probabilities at each step. If there were four incidents, the susceptible (disease-free) partner could be infected at any one of the four incidents. We could estimate the probability of being infected by adding up all the paths through the tree in which the organism ends up being transmitted to the partner at least once. This is somewhat simplified by truncating the tree at

282

the first point of successful transmission. However, the calculation is drastically simplified by realizing that the overall probability of infection is one minus the probability the partner is not infected and the only sequence that would leave the susceptible partner uninfected at the end of the year would be the combination of 100 events in which the infection was not transmitted.

The probability of 100 incidents without transmission is the product of the probabilities of the individual outcomes. So if the couple is still discordant after 100 exposures, the probability of that occurring is $(1-Pi)^{100}$.

In the case of HIV or HSV, the probability of infection after 100 exposures in monogamous discordant couples has been observed to be about 10%. Thus, the probability of not being infected is 90% and this is equal to $(1-Pi)^{100}$.

Solving for Pi reveals that the probability of being infected in one incident under these circumstances is about 0.00105

Tree diagram for probability of infection from four exposures (picture this with 100 branches):

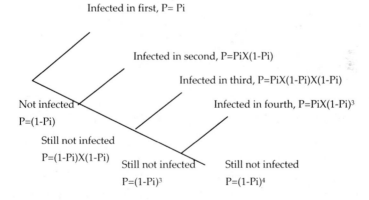

Infected in first, P= Pi

Infected in second, P=PiX(1-Pi)

Infected in third, P=PiX(1-Pi)X(1-Pi)

Infected in fourth, P=PiX(1-Pi)^3

Not infected
P=(1-Pi)

Still not infected
P=(1-Pi)X(1-Pi)

Still not infected
P=(1-Pi)^3

Still not infected
P=(1-Pi)^4

The fact that this is a binomial model rather than a linear additive model means that the probability of being infected after 1000 exposures (which might be about ten years) is not certainty, but, rather, about 65%. The effect of condoms, properly used could be a reduction of as much as 90%, so there would be a pretty low probability of transmitting the HIV even after ten years.

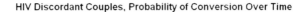
HIV Discordant Couples, Probability of Conversion Over Time

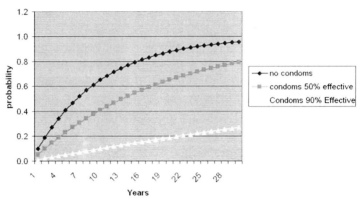

An unsophisticated observer might expect that with a Pi of 1/1000, within ten years, there is a 100% probability of infections and there is no point in taking precautions. In fact, here is a chart showing probability of infection as modified by use of condoms, which are variously estimated to be between 50% and 90% effective, depending on the STD and consistency of use.

As you can see, probability of infection after a ten year relationship is substantially less than 100%, and use of condoms, even at the lowest estimated reliability is a worthwhile proposition. You shouldn't necessarily assume that someone who has been in risky relationships for a number of years is infected—especially if they have consistently followed risk-reducing procedures.

This simplified version is substantially hampered by the fact that Pi is affected drastically by a number of other factors, such as stage in the infection, type of sex, presence of other STDs—especially ulcerating STDs, and the influence of sexual network configurations in multi-partner circumstances.

284

Effect of sexual network configuration on dissemination of STDs

Persistence of sexually transmitted infections depends on a reproductive number greater than one, and is only possible when relationships involve more than two people.

However, "monogamy" is a relative concept. It might be more realistic to think of monogamists as "serial monogamists" who may be involved in more than one relationship over a lifetime, but it is only one at a time and there is little or no overlap in time. Almost all marriages suffer divorce or death of one spouse, in which case there is usually a second relationship for the survivors. However, in serial monogamy—i.e. involving multiple partners with no back and forth—there is usually adequate separation in time so that any infections acquired in the first become apparent or diagnosable before entering into the next relationship. Awareness may lead to cure, when possible, or treatment or other precautions to reduce probability of passing it forward. There is also the important fact that it isn't possible to communicate a future infection back to past partners.

Pairs that are consonant, either in being infected or not, remain so in a monogamous relationship. Pairs that are dissonant may eventually become consonant, but there is no opportunity for further infection.

Thus, Concurrent multiple partner relationships in which one or more partner goes back and forth between two or more other people are more effective in disseminating STDs.

The efficacy of temporal overlaps in transmitting disease
depends on configurations of networks and intervals between relations, as well as the nature of the disease:

- **Duration of the infection**
- **Time to Patency, and**
- **Stage of infection effects on potency**

Most people are somewhat discriminating in sexual contacts. This results in social compartmentation or segregation of social groups that provides insulation or "firewalls" to impede the progression of an infection throughout the whole population.

At the same time, a tighter web of interactions within smaller groups may lead to a more effective permeation within that subgroup.

As far back as the 1970's (St John and Curran, 1978) noted that repetitive infections in a small percentage (3-7%) of infected persons accounted for about 30% of the caseload of some gonorrhea clinics. This led to the notion of "core groups" that maintain a pool of infection so that it is difficult to eradicate in the overall population. Core groups include high-risk behavior groups such as MSM, IDU and commercial sex workers.

When people consort with others who have like characteristics, this is called an *assortative* interaction. For example, people with high sexual activity patterns consort with others who are also very sexually active. Groups may also be sexually segregated by characteristics such as ethnicity, socioeconomic class, or age.

Dissortative interaction refers to partnering with people from other groups, or reaching across groups. Theoretical studies show that assortative interactions lead to more rapid initial spread of an STD within a subgroup, but a smaller extent of the overall epidemic, as it is limited in passing to other compartments. Dissortative patterns, on the other hand, give a slower start, but a broader dissemination, and an ultimately larger epidemic.

Several authors have speculated that the higher rates of STDs in some ethnic/cultural groups are a result of sexual and behavioral segregation (Liljeros, *et al.*, 2003).

Even people with relatively low risk behaviors, although following a strict one-partner rule, may be at substantial risk if they are partnered with someone who is not so strict and makes connections with other parties at high risk of infection. Often, the other partner—say, a straying husband—in the interests of discretion, may seek a liaison with a sex worker or other anonymous connection with someone who has random relationships that go across groups.

Likewise consider the ostensibly faithful Senator who indulges clandestine bisexuality through anonymous random connections in gay bars or bathhouses. Attempts to maintain anonymity may result in relationship patterns that are more random with respect to risk groups and other strata.

Some have argued that reduction of social stigma and legalization of prostitution reduces spread of disease because legal prostitutes are frequently tested and treated if necessary. This may be true for curable diseases such as gonorrhea, especially since gonorrhea is unlikely to be noticed in an infected female in the absence of testing.

However, the time of highest infectiousness for HIV, for example, has been shown to be in the early stages of infection before antibodies are detectable.

Cultural subsets with random relationships across strata provide a particularly potent conduit for transmission of infections across groups that might otherwise be insulated. This has led to the concept of a "sexual bridge" between compartments and the location of bridge connections is especially important in the rate of spread of an STI. For example, envision two different configurations of 8 different subjects who interact with each other or each others' partners in a sexual network (diagram from Wohlfeier and Potterat, 2003):

Each configuration has a total of eight people connected in nine relationships: six have only two partners, two have three each. However, the effectiveness of transmission will be much more effective in configuration B than in configuration A. In network B, six of the seven susceptible parties can be infected in only two steps from the person at the left end. In Network A, it would take 4 steps to achieve the same penetration. As well, transmission can be blocked from half the network by severing only one relationship in A, but three interventions are required to interrupt the course of transmission in network B.

Anything that compartmentalizes subgroups is a barrier to propagation. One very interesting compartmentalization that might use more thoughtful exploration is the concept of "age appropriateness" of relationships.

As noted earlier, infections which are not fatal but are not curable would be expected to accumulate as people have more exposure over time just due to more experience. Certainly more active younger people could have more cumulative exposures than the average senior citizen, but other things being equal, older means more likely to have been infected. This has been noted for CMV and HSV-2.

Although it might seem excessively intrusive and pretty silly to promote mores related to age-assortative ("age-appropriate") relationships, the discussion by Morris (1997) leads to some interesting thoughts.

Assortative age-matching has been shown to result in lower risk of exposure for younger cohorts, and MSM with older partners can be a leading edge for introducing infections in younger groups (Morris et al., 1995, Service and Blower, 1995). Morris (1997) concludes:

"In heterosexual partnerships, such age asymmetry is common. and the pairing of older men with younger women is often found. This virtually ensures a strong intergenerational chain of transmission: a high prevalence cohort of older men infects the newly active cohort of young women, who eventually pass it on to their male age-peers, who become the next cohort of older men, and so on."

One could envision the aging of infected cohorts as an infective pool traveling down a closed pipeline to extinction as the cohort eventually died out. Although there would be some mixing at the interface of older and younger groups, minimization of any "backwash effect" would eventually lead to the extinction of the infection. Age dissortative relationships provide a backwash effect by shunting the infection back into an earlier part of the pipeline and preventing extinction.

Implications for Intervention

Civil libertarians have argued that it is wrong to interfere with a citizen's private sexual behavior and that activities such as prostitution and drug abuse are "victimless crimes." This attitude might be epitomized in the famous expression, sometimes attributed to Lady Astor, "do anything you want, just don't scare the horses."

It is argued that legalization of drugs and prostitution would improve the situation because it would introduce regulation, testing and, of course, tax revenues.

Public messages intended to reduce risky behavior have focused on risk to the perpetrator rather than on risk to innocent partners (although there has been some mention of potential damage to unborn children). One might conclude that if you are willing to bear the risk, then it's your business what you do. Introduction of a *quid pro quo* sometimes generates an attitude that "if you are willing to pay the price, then it is moral to indulge in the behavior."

Increasing awareness of the "down low" phenomenon among MSM and IDU has added momentum to legislative action making it a crime to knowingly infect another person with HIV, and there have been successful civil lawsuits against parties who knew of their STD infections but did not notify partners of the risk.

It's clear that the most effective opportunities for intervention are with core and bridge groups. Promotion of monogamy and discouragement of random pairing are important.

Multiple concurrent relationships should be discouraged by emphasizing the responsibility to protect innocent partners by a strict serial monogamy—defined as allowing a long enough between relationships to allow for any infections to become apparent and treated or cured, if possible. Programs should publicize the time to patency, diagnostic issues and infectiousness related to stage of the diseases. Partners have a right to be aware of their risks.

Influence of positive social organizations

Small group activity in churches and other social organizations that encourage assortative pairing among low risk individuals is likely to reduce the occurrence of innocent victims, and provide a barrier to bridging from high risk core groups.

Although not clearly an ethical issue, these same organizations could support the benefits of age-assortative pairing by recognizing other benefits such as stage-of-life compatibility regarding such issues as desire to have children, career goals, and mutual comfort and support at later stages of life, and death.

Legislation

Prostitution is not clearly a "victimless crime" as prostitutes, more often than not, are collaborating in a violation of the rights of their clients' other partners. The argument for legalization, testing and taxing is invalidated by the recognition that some infections are most virulent in the early stages before they are detectable.

Focus on the ethical issue in prevention programs

Perhaps media programs to discourage high risk behavior should focus less on the risk to the individual (which is subject to rationalization) and more on the ethical issue of unfairly exposing innocent partners—particularly "loved-ones"—to consequences they don't deserve.

See std-statistics.com and socialsimulations.com for details on calculations shown in this chapter and continuing work on mathematical models on the spread of infectious diseases and other social issues.

References and Bibliography:

ACLU (2004) State Criminal Statutes on HIV Transmission – 2004 This chart, updated in 2004, is based on earlier compilations by the ACLU's National Prison Project and Lambda Legal Defense and Education Fund, ,part of the Lesbian and Gay Rights Project/AIDS project. At ACLU.ORG

ANDERSON, ROY M. PhD, FRS; GARNETT, GEOFFREY P. PhD, BSc (2000) Mathematical Models of the Transmission and Control of Sexually Transmitted Diseases. Sexually Transmitted Diseases. 27(10):636-643, November 2000.).

Blower, S (2004) Modeling the Genital Herpes Epidemic, Herpes 11 Supplement 3

CDC (2004) The *HIV/AIDS Surveillance Report*.Vol 16, 2004

CDC (2005) 2004 STD Surveillance Report, Sept 2005

CDC (2005) Hepatitis Surveillance Report No. 60, Sept. 2005

Corey L (2004) Clinical Tools for Preventing Sexual Transmission of Genital Herpes, Medscape Infectious Diseases 6(1), 2004

Fleming DT, McQuillan GM, Johnson RE, Nahmias AJ, Aral SO, Lee FK, St. Louis ME. Herpes Simplex Virus Type 2 in the United States, 1976 to 1994. NEJM 1997; 16:1105-1111.

Gray,RH, Maria J Wawer, Ron Brookmeyer, Nelson K Sewankambo, David Serwadda, Fred Wabwire-Mangen, Tom Lutalo, Xianbin Li, Thomas vanCott, Thomas C Quinn, and the Rakai Project Team (2001) Probability of HIV-1 transmission per coital act in monogamous, heterosexual, HIV-1-discordant couples in Rakai, Uganda THE LANCET Vol 357:1149 April 14, 2001

Levin BR, Bull JJ and Stewart FM (2001) Epidemiology, Evolution and Future of the HIV/AIDS Pandemic, Presentation from the 2000 Emerging Infectious Diseases Conference, Vol 7, No 3 Supplement Jun 2001

Liljeros, Fredrik a,b, Christofer R. Edling b,c, Luis A. Nunes Amaral (2003) Sexual networks: implications for the transmission of sexually transmitted infections, Microbes and Infection 5:189-196

Mertz GJ, Benedetti J, Ashley R Selke SA, Corey L.,(1992) Risk factors for the sexual transmission of genital herpes, Ann Intern Med 1992 Feb 1;116(3):197-202

World Bank Group (1997) "Confronting AIDS: Public Priorities in a Global Epidemic" is a World Bank report published in November 1997 by the Oxford University Press

Morris M. (1997) Sexual networks and HIV. AIDS. 1997;11:S209-216

Morris M,Dean L: Social and sexual networks: their role in the spread of HIV among young gay men. AIDS Educ Prev 1995, 7:S24-S35

NIAD Staff (2001) Scientific Evidence on Condom Effectiveness for Sexually Transmitted Disease (STD) Prevention, Workshop Summary, June 12-13,2000

NIH (1995) Infectious Disease Testing for Blood Transfusion, NIH Consensus Statement Volume 13, Number 1 Jan 1995

Service S, Blower S: HIV Transmission in sexual networks: an empirical analysis, Proc R Soc Lond B Biol Sci 1995, 260:237-244.

St. John R, Curran J, Epidemiology of Gonorrhea, Sex Transm Dis 1978 5:81-82

Wohlfeier D and Potterat J, UCSF April 2003 Fact Sheet #50E, Center for AIDS Prevention Studies at the University of California San Francisco

Other Books

Books from Science & Humanities Press

HOW TO TRAVEL—A Guidebook for Persons with a Disability – Fred Rosen (1997) ISBN 1-888725-05-2, 5½ X 8¼, 120 pp, $9.95 18-point large print edition (1998) ISBN 1-888725-17-6 7X8, 120 pp, $19.95

HOW TO TRAVEL in Canada—A Guidebook for A Visitor with a Disability – Fred Rosen (2000) ISBN 1-888725-26-5, 5½X8¼, 180 pp, $14.95 MacroPrintBooks™ edition (2001) ISBN 1-888725-30-3 7X8, 16 pt, 200 pp, $19.95

How to travel to and in Britain & Northern Ireland : a guidebook for visitors with a disability – Fred Rosen (2006) ISBN 1-888725-47-8, 5½X8¼, 190 pp, $14.95 MacroPrintBooks™ edition (2001) ISBN 1-888725-48-6, 7X8, 16 pt, 200 pp, $19.95

AVOIDING Attendants from HELL: A Practical Guide to Finding, Hiring & Keeping Personal Care Attendants 2nd Edn—June Price, (2002), accessible plastic spiral bind, ISBN 1-888725-72-9 8¼X10½, 125 pp, $16.95, School/library edition (2002) ISBN 1-888725-60-5, 8¼X6½, 200 pp, $18.95

Spiritual Journeys in Prayer and Song with music CD, Reverend Peter Unger, 2006. Short Christian meditations with accompanying songs on CD ISBN 1-59630-009-4 (regular print edition) 5½X8¼, 185 pp, $24.95 ISBN 1-59630-010-8 MacroPrintBooks Large Print edition, 16 point type $29.95

The Bridge Never Crossed—A Survivor's Search for Meaning. Captain George A. Burk (1999) The inspiring story of George Burk, lone survivor of a military{ XE "military" } plane crash, who overcame extensive burn injuries to earn a presidential award and become a highly successful motivational speaker. ISBN 1-888725-16-8, 5½X8¼, 170 pp, illustrated. $16.95 MacroPrintBooks™ Edition (1999) ISBN 1-888725-28-1 $24.95

Value Centered Leadership—A Survivor's Strategy for Personal and Professional Growth—Captain George A. Burk (2004) Principles of Leadership & Total Quality Management applied to all aspects of living. ISBN 1-888725-59-1, 5½X8¼, 120 pp, $16.95

Paul the Peddler or The Fortunes of a Young Street Merchant—Horatio Alger, jr A Classic reprinted in accessible large type, (1998 MacroPrintBooks™ reprint in 24-point type) ISBN 1-888725-02-8, 8¼X10½, 276 pp, $16.95

The Wisdom of Father Brown—G.K. Chesterton (2000) A Classic collection of detective stories reprinted in accessible 22-point type ISBN 1-888725-27-3 8¼X10½, 276 pp, $18.95

24-point Gospel—The Big News for Today – The Gospel according to Matthew, Mark, Luke & John (KJV) in 24-point type is about 1/3 inch high. Now, people with visual disabilities like macular degeneration can still use this important reference. "Giant print" books are usually 18 pt. or less ISBN 1-888725-11-7, 8¼X10½, 512 pp, $24.95

Buttered Side Down—Short Stories by Edna Ferber (BeachHouse Books reprint 2000) A classic collection of stories by the beloved author of Showboat, Giant, and Cimarron. ISBN 1-888725-43-5, 5½X8¼, 190 pp, $12.95 MacroPrintBooks™ Edition (2000) ISBN 1-888725-40-0 7X8¼,16 pt, 240 pp $18.95

The Four Million: The Gift of the Magi & other favorites. Life in New York City around 1900—O. Henry. MacroPrintBooks™ reprint (2001) ISBN 1-888725-41-9 7X8¼, 16 pt, 270 pp $18.95; ISBN 1-888725-03-6, 8¼X10½, 22 pt, 300pp, $22.95

Bar-20: Hopalong Cassidy's Rustler Roundup— Clarence Mulford (reprint 2000). Classical Western Tale. Not the TV version. ISBN 1-888725-34-6 5½X8¼, 223 pp, $12.95 Macro-

PrintBooks™ edition ISBN 1-888725-42-7, 8¼X6½, 16 pt, 385pp, $18.95

Nursing Home – Ira Eaton, PhD, (1997) You will be moved and disturbed by this novel. ISBN 1-888725-01-X, 5½X8¼, 300 pp, $12.95 MacroPrintBooks™ edition (1999) ISBN 1-888725-23-0,8¼X10½, 16 pt, 330 pp, $18.95

Perfect Love-A Novel by Mary Harvatich (2000) Love born in an orphanage endures ISBN 1-888725-29-X 5½X8¼, 200 pp, $12.95 MacroPrintBooks™ edition (2000) ISBN 1-888725-15-X, 8¼X10½, 16 pt, 200 pp, $18.95

The Essential Simply Speaking Gold – Susan Fulton, (1998) How to use IBM's popular speech recognition package for dictation rather than keyboarding. Dozens of screen shots and illustrations. ISBN 1-888725-08-7 8¼ X8, 124 pp, $18.95

Begin Dictation Using ViaVoice Gold -2nd Edition– Susan Fulton, (1999), Covers ViaVoice 98 and other versions of IBM's popular continuous speech recognition package for dictation rather than keyboarding. Over a hundred screen shots and illustrations. ISBN 1-888725-22-2, 8¼X8, 260 pp, $28.95

Ropes and Saddles—Andy Polson (2001) Cowboy (and other) poems by Andy Polson. Reminiscences of the Wyoming poet. ISBN 1-888725-39-7, 5½ X 8¼, 100 pp, $9.95

Tales from the Woods of Wisdom—(book I)— Richard Tichenor (2000) In a spirit someplace between The Wizard of Oz and The Celestine Prophecy, this is more than a childrens' fable of life in the deep woods. ISBN 1-888725-37-0, 5½X8¼, 185 pp, $16.95 MacroPrintBooks™ edition (2001) ISBN 1-888725-50-8 6X8¼, 16 pt, 270 pp $24.95

Me and My Shadows—Shadow Puppet Fun for Kids of All Ages—Elizabeth Adams, Revised Edition by Dr. Bud Banis

(2000) A thoroughly illustrated guide to the art of shadow puppet entertainment using tools that are always at hand wherever you go. A perfect gift for children and adults. ISBN 1-888725-44-3, 7X8¼, 67 pp, 12.95 MacroPrintBooks™ edition (2002) ISBN 1-888725-78-8 8½X11 lay-flat spiral, 18 pt, 67 pp, $16.95

Eudora Light™ v 3.0 Manual (Qualcomm 1996) ISBN 1-888725-20-6½, extensively illustrated. 135 pp, 5½ X 8¼, $9.95

MamaSquad! (2001) Hilarious novel by Clarence Wall about what happens when a group of women from a retirement home get tangled up in Army Special Forces. ISBN 1-888725-13-3 5½ X8¼, 200 pp, $14.95 MacroPrintBooks™ edition (2001) ISBN 1-888725-14-1 8¼X6½ 16 pt, 300 pp, $24.95

Virginia Mayo—The Best Years of My Life (2002) Autobiography of film star Virginia Mayo as told to LC Van Savage. From her early days in Vaudeville and the Muny in St Louis to the dozens of hit motion pictures, with dozens of photographs. ISBN 1-888725-53-2, 5½ X 8¼, 200 pp, $16.95

The Job—Eric Whitfield (2001) A story of self-discovery in the context of the death of a grandfather.. A book to read and share in times of change and Grieving. ISBN 1-888725-68-0, 5½ X 8¼, 100 pp, $12.95 MacroPrintBooks™ edition (2001) ISBN 1-888725-69-9, 8¼X6½, 18 pt, 150 pp, $18.95

Plague Legends: from the Miasmas of Hippocrates to the Microbes of Pasteur-Socrates Litsios D.Sc. (2001) Medical progress from early history through the 19th Century in understanding origins and spread of contagious disease. A thorough but readable and enlightening history of medicine. Illustrated, Bibliography, Index ISBN 1-888725-33-8, 6¼X8¼, 250pp, $24.95

The Cut—John Evans (2003). Football, Mystery and Mayhem in a highschool setting by John Evans ISBN: 1-888725-82-6 5½ X 8¼, 100 pp $14.95 **MacroPrintBooks**™ edition (2003) 16 pt. ISBN: 1-888725-83-4 $24.95

Sexually Transmitted Diseases—Symptoms, Diagnosis, Treatment, Prevention-2nd Edition – NIAID Staff, Assembled and Edited by R.J.Banis, PhD, (2006) Teacher friendly —free to copy for education. Illustrated with more than 50 photographs of lesions, ISBN 1-888725-58-3, 8¼X6½, 290 pp, $18.95

The Stress Myth -Serge Doublet, PhD (2000) A thorough examination of the concept that 'stress' is the source of unexplained afflictions. Debunking mysticism, psychologist Serge Doublet reviews the history of other concepts such as 'demons', 'humors', 'hysteria' and 'neurasthenia' that had been placed in this role in the past, and provides an alternative approach for more success in coping with life's challenges. ISBN 1-888725-36-2, 5½X8¼, 280 pp, $24.95

Behind the Desk Workout – Joan Guccione, OTR/C, CHT (1997) ISBN 1-888725-00-1, Reduce risk of injury by exercising regularly at your desk. Over 200 photos and illustrations. (lay-flat spiral) 8¼X10½, 120 pp, $34.95 Paperback edition, (2000) ISBN 1-888725-25-7 $24.95

Copyright Issues for Librarians, Teachers & Authors–R.J. Banis, PhD, (Ed). 2nd Edn (2001) Protecting your rights, respecting others'. Information condensed from the Library of Congress, copyright registration forms. ISBN 1-888725-62-1, 5¼X8¼, 60 pp, booklet. $4.95

Rhythm of the Sea —Shari Cohen (2001). Delightful collection of heartwarming stories of life relationships set in the context of oceans and lakes. Shari Cohen is a popular author of Womens' magazine articles and contributor to the

Chicken Soup for the Soul series. ISBN 1-888725-55-9, 8X6.5 150 pp, $14.95 MacroPrintBooks™ edition (2001) ISBN 1-888725-63-X, 8¼X6½, 16 pt, 250 pp, $24.95

To Norma Jeane With Love, Jimmie -Jim Dougherty as told to LC Van Savage (2001) ISBN 1-888725-51-6 The sensitive and touching story of Jim Dougherty's teenage bride who later became Marilyn Monroe. Dozens of photographs. "The Marilyn Monroe book of the year!" As seen on TV. 5½X8¼, 200 pp, $16.95 MacroPrintBooks™ edition ISBN 1-888725-52-4, 8¼X6½, 16 pt, 290pp, $24.95

Riverdale Chronicles—Charles F. Rechlin (2003). Life, living and character studies in the setting of the Riverdale Golf Club by Charles F. Rechlin 5½ X 8¼, 100 pp ISBN: 1-888725-84-2 $14.95 **MacroPrintBooks**™ edition (2003) 16 pt. 8¼X6½, 16 pt, 350 pp ISBN: 1-888725-85-0 $24.95

Winners and Losers--Charles F. Rechlin (2005). a collection of humorous short stories portraying misadventures of attorneys, stock brokers, and others in the Urban workplace. ISBN 1-59630-002-7 BeachHouse Books Edition $14.95 ISBN 1-59630-003-5 MacroPrintBooks Edition (large print) $24.95

Bloodville — Don Bullis (2002) Fictional adaptation of the Budville, NM murders by New Mexico crime historian, Don Bullis. 5½ X 8¼, 350 pp ISBN: 1-888725-75-3 $14.95 **Macro-PrintBooks**™ edition (2003) 16 pt. 8¼X11 460pp ISBN: 1-888725-76-1 $24.95

Ellos Pasaron por Aqui — 99 New Mexicans and a Few Other Folks (2005) compilation of old-time stories illustrates how the Wild West really was during New Mexico's frontier era. ISBN 1-888725-92-3, 6½ X 8¼, 350 pp, $16.95 Macro-PrintBooks™ edition ISBN 1-888725-93-1, 350pp 8¼ X 11, 16 pt, $24.95

Republican or Democrat? (2005) Moses Sanchez, who describes himself as "a Black Hispanic" thinks for himself, questions the stereotypes, examines the facts and makes his own decision. Early Editions Books ISBN 1-888725-32-X 5½X8¼, 176pp pp, $14.95

50 Things You Didn't Learn in School–But Should Have: Little known facts that still affect our world today (2005) by John Naese, . ISBN 1-888725-49-4, 5½X8¼, 200 pp, illustrated. $16.95

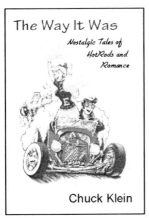

The Way It Was

Nostalgic Tales of HotRods and Romance

Chuck Klein

The Way It Was-- Nostalgic Tales of Hotrods and Romance Chuck Klein (2003) Series of hotrod stories by author of Circa 1957 in collaboration with noted illustrator Bill Lutz BeachHouse Books edition 5½ X 8¼, 200 pp ISBN: 1-888725-86-9 $14.95

MacroPrintBooks™ edition (2003) 16 pt. 8¼X6½, 350pp ISBN: 1-888725-87-7 $24.95

Route 66 books by Michael Lund

Growing Up on Route 66 —Michael Lund (2000) ISBN 1-888725-31-1 Novel evoking fond memories of what it was like to grow up alongside "America's Highway" in 20th Century Missouri. (Trade paperback) 5½ X8¼, 260 pp, $14.95 **MacroPrintBooks**™ edition (2001) ISBN 1-888725-45-1 8¼X6½, 16 pt, 330 pp, $24.95

Route 66 Kids —Michael Lund (2002) ISBN 1-888725-70-2 Sequel to *Growing Up on Route 66*, continuing memories of what it was like to grow up alongside "America's Highway" in 20th Century Missouri. (Trade paperback) 5½ X8¼, 270 pp, $14.95 **MacroPrintBooks**™ edition (2002) ISBN 1-888725-71-0 8¼X6½, 16 pt, 350 pp, $24.95

A Left-hander on Route 66--Michael Lund (2003) ISBN 1-888725-88-5. Twenty years after the fact, left-hander Hugh Noone appeals a wrongful conviction that detoured him from "America's Main Street" and put him in jail. But revealing the details of the past and effecting a resolution of his case mean a dramatic rearrangement of his world, including troubled relationships with three women: Linda Roy, Patty Simpson, and Karen Murphy. (Trade paperback) 5½ X8¼, 270 pp, $14.95 **MacroPrintBooks**™ edition (2002) ISBN 1-888725-89-3 8¼X6½, 16 pt, 350 pp, $24.95

Miss Route 66--Michael Lund (2004) ISBN 1-888725-96-6. In the fourth novel of Michael Lund's Route 66 Novel Series, Susan Bell tells the story of her candidacy in Fairfield, Missouri's annual beauty contest. Now married and with teenage children in St. Louis, she recounts her youthful adventure in this small town along "America's Highway." At the same time, she plans a return to Fairfield in order to right injustices she feels were done to some young contestants in the Miss Route 66 Pageant. (Trade paperback) 5½ X8¼, 260 pp, $14.95 **MacroPrintBooks**™ edition (2004) ISBN 1-888725-97-4 8¼X6½, 16 pt, 350 pp, $24.95

AudioBook on CD-- Miss Route 66 ISBN: 1-888725-12-5 by Michael Lund unabridged 5 CD's --7 Hours running time. $24.95

Route 66 Spring-- Michael Lund (2004) ISBN: 1-888725-98-2. The lives of four young Missourians are changed when a bottle comes to the surface of one of the state's many natural springs. Inside is a letter written by a girl a dozen years after the end of the Civil War. Lucy Rivers Johns ' epistle contains a sad story of family failure and a powerful plea for help.

This message from the last century crystallizes the individual frustrations of Janet Masters, Freddy Sills, Louis Clark, and Roberta Green, another group of Route 66 kids. Their response to the past charts a bold path into the future, a path inspired by the Mother Road itself. (Trade paperback) 5½ X8¼, 270 pp, $14.95. MacroPrintBooks™ edition (2002) ISBN 1-888725-99-0. 8¼X6½, 16 pt, 350 pp, $24.95.

Route 66 to Vietnam Michael Lund (2004) ISBN 1-59630-000-0 This novel takes characters from earlier works in the Route 66 Novel Series farther west than Los Angeles, official destination of the famous highway, Route 66. Mark Landon and Billy Rhodes find the values they grew up on challenged by America's role in Southeast Asia. But elements of their upbringing represented by the Mother Road also sustain them in ways they could never have anticipated. . (Trade paperback) 5½ X8¼, 270 pp, $14.95. MacroPrintBooks™ edition (2004) ISBN 1-59630-001-9. 8¼X6½, 16 pt, 350 pp, $24.95.

Journey to a Closed City with the International Executive Service Corps—Russell R. Miller (2004) ISBN 1-888725-94-X, Describes the adventures of a retired executive volunteering with the senior citizens' equivalent of the Peace Corp as he applies his professional skills in a former Iron Curtain city emerging into the dawn of a new economy.This book is essential reading for anyone approaching retirement who is interested in opportunities to exercise skills to "do good" during expense-paid travel to intriguing locations. Journey to A Closed City should also appeal to armchair travelers eager to explore far-off corners of the world in our rapidly-evolving global community. paperback, 5½X8¼,270pp,$16.95 **MacroPrintBooks**™ edition (2004) ISBN 1-888725-94-8, 8¼X6½, 18 pt, 150 pp, $24.95

Inaugural Addresses: Presidents of the United States from George Washington to 2008 -3rd Edition– Robert J. Banis, PhD, CMA, Ed. (2005) ISBN 1-59630-004-3, 7X8½, 400pp., extensively illustrated, includes election statistics, Vice-presidents, principal opponents, coupons for update supplements for the upcoming election $18.95

Science & Humanities Press

Publishes fine books under the imprints:

- Science & Humanities Press
- BeachHouse Books
- MacroPrint Books
- Heuristic Books
- Early Editions Books

Our books are guaranteed:

If a book has a defect, or doesn't hold up under normal use, or if you are unhappy in any way with one of our books, we are interested to know about it and will replace it and credit reasonable return shipping costs. Products with publisher defects (i.e., books with missing pages, etc.) may be returned at any time without authorization. However, we request that you describe the problem, to help us to continuously improve.

Some recent books by R. Banis

Sexually Transmitted Diseases—Symptoms, Diagnosis, Treatment, Prevention-2nd Edition – NIAID Staff, Assembled and Edited by R.J.Banis, PhD, (2006) Teacher friendly —free to copy for education. Illustrated with more than 70 figures and photographs of lesions, ISBN 1-888725-58-3, 8¼X5½, 290 pp, $18.95

Youth Risk Behavior Survey with Student Guide for Statistical Analysis in EXCEL, R. J. Banis, PhD & Centers for Disease Control Staff (2006) ISBN 1-888725-24-9 Heuristic Books, 8½X11, spiral bound, 250 pp, $28.95

Order Form

Item	Each	Quantity	Amount
Missouri (only) sales tax			
Priority Shipping			$4.00
	Total		
Name			
Address			

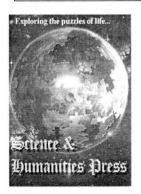

Science & Humanities Press

PO Box 7151

Chesterfield, MO 63006-7151

(636) 394-4950
sciencehumanitiespress.com